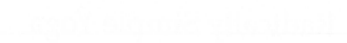

Radically Simple Yoga

For Now

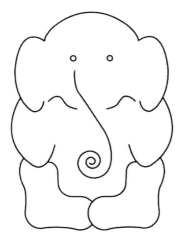

To all those who take the courage to practice a yoga that is
simple, authentic and personally empowering.

Published by Akhuratha Publishing.

First Edition

© David Dodd 2016

A catalogue record for this book is available from the British Library.

ISBN 978-0-9935348-0-5

Cover Illustration: Eva Thomassen

Cover Design: Chris Kerslake

Interior Illustrations: David Dodd & Chris Kerslake

Printed and bound by IngramSpark.

www.radicallysimpleyoga.com

Contents

About This Book

Radically Simple Yoga

This book presents an approach to yoga that is both radical and simple. It goes to the root of the messages underlying the two most widely acclaimed yoga texts, the Yoga Sutras of Patanjali and the Bhagavad Gita, and frames these within the context of the shifts and challenges of our modern world. *Radically Simple Yoga* presents old wisdom in the language of our times for the practice of yoga on our mats and for taking our yoga off our mats and into our worlds.

Radically Simple Yoga steps back from, and cuts through, the differences of tradition and style to the essence of our approach to yoga practice. It moves beyond the interests of competing yoga traditions old and new and those from the East and from the West; traditions that often both simplify yoga into a commodity and make yoga appear more complicated than it is. This book focuses our attention on an inner approach to practice that is applicable within all traditions and styles.

Radically Simple Yoga explores how our inner approach to practice can support us in growing connection. It explores how our inner approach to practice supports us in moving first beyond the illusions of separation we experience on the inside and then those we experience between inside and outside. This book expands on the radically simple message of yoga that all is connected and that it is above all our inner approach to practice that empowers us to realise and to act from wholeness.

For Now

When we focus our attention on our inner approach to yoga we empower our practice and our selves in ways that serve the shifting of our times: a shifting away from a worldview of separation and towards one of connection. *Radically Simple Yoga* explores how yoga grows our individual and communal agency - our ability to act and to have effect - from the perspective of connection. It explores how yoga does this in a way that works from the inside out and manifests unrestricted by the imposition of external codes.

This book presents nothing new: yoga has always in essence been an inner practice, and the heart of yoga has always been connection and, through connection, empowerment. With yoga's explosion in popularity over the past few decades, and in particular the focus on yoga for well-being and relaxation, our attention has been drawn to methods for the physical postures. As more and more of us wake up to the power and potential of yoga it will be our inner approach to practice, and the connection with our inner source of peace, joy and love, and of strength, purpose and creativity, that supports us as we learn and grow as individuals and as communities.

Seven Inner Props

Radically Simple Yoga offers seven inner props - or attitude skills - for making our inner approach to yoga real. The props are introduced at the end of the first section of each chapter and the final section of each chapter explores the prop in the context of our mat-based practice and our lives off the mat. Whilst we will explore these one by one, these props are much more akin to a virtuous circle, a mutually reinforcing interdependent set of skills.

Radically Simple Yoga is not another brand or form of yoga: these inner props are not set in stone and there are no seven laws of inner practice. These props are offered simply to give direction and structure for our exploration towards wholeness and, just like the props for yoga posture in class, we may need to modify, drop them or find others. When it comes to yoga as life there is only one rule: our full undivided participation is required - we are here to experience and to engage fully in that experience.

To practice yoga in a way that is radical and simple is to embark on reclaiming our agency and to engage in a subtle yet deep act of political disruption. Sooner or later our practice brings us to those two questions at the heart of the shifting of our times: who am I, and how am I going to spend my time here? When we engage with these two questions our practice teaches us that they have, at their root, one answer: an answer that cannot be grasped by mind and an answer that we each embody in our own sweet way.

About the Author

David Dodd is currently entangled in a persona play to bring empowerment to people at work and through yoga. Beyond his own experience David has no particular qualifications to write anything meaningful about life in general or yoga specifically. After living for 20 years in the Netherlands, David has recently moved to the UK.

Do your practice. Enjoy the ride!

1. Radically Simple Yoga

Yoga is an experiential system: to reap the benefits we have to practice. Whatever forms our practice and our motivation take it is how we practice that makes it yoga. Skill in how we practice begins with growing our awareness.

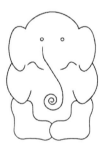

Doorways to Yoga

Yoga rocks! Yoga has rocked in India for thousands of years. Way back in time yoga rocked the wild men and women of the shamanic traditions gathered around their fires, the recluses of the Himalayas sitting solitary in their lofty caves and the tantric practitioners hidden deep in their forest ashrams. Yoga rocked the Brahman priests in their temples and kings in their palaces. With revived interest over the past century groups as diverse as the fresh-faced recruits to the Indian army and the well-oiled bodies of the Indian body-building community have taken up yoga.

From that revived interest the party has come to the West and the West has joined the party. We have joined the party with a bang and embraced yoga with open arms. Every day tens of millions of us roll out our mats in yoga studios, sports clubs and at home to practice. Yoga classes in the studio around the corner, in the downtown gym, and online have opened the doors to many. They have made the immediate benefits of stress-reduction and improved well-being accessible. The West has made yoga its own and we want more.

Yoga is here now and we all find our own way into yoga - we each have our own doorway. We all have our reasons for taking up yoga practice. In the West today many come to yoga motivated by a desire for health and well-being. We may want to lose weight, to gain flexibility, and to build strength. We may be motivated by stories told to us by friends who are already practicing, or by the broad and well-founded reputation yoga has for achieving results, or by the slim and toned bodies on the covers of the yoga magazines. Many more of us come to yoga to de-stress. We may be looking to loosen that tight feeling somewhere deep down in our belly or up around our heart. We may want to free up our shoulders, or quieten down our non-stop minds. We come to attend to the varying ways in which stress manifests in us. Then there are those of us who come to yoga to address specific dis-ease; we may suffer from an acute or chronic complaint for which we seek healing.

Yet more of us come to yoga in search of spiritual or personal development: we come to reconnect with our self, to find a sense of purpose or to infuse spirit into our being and our life. We may find yoga, or yoga finds us, at a time of personal crisis, at a time when we have taken a big hit to our worldview. For many of us this is a time when our sense of aloneness, our sense of separation from both our selves and those around us, is intense. A time when from one perspective we seem to be struggling, whilst from another we are just one step nearer to freedom. Or our reason may be something else altogether: how we find our way to yoga is both quintessentially important and utterly irrelevant.

Practice! Practice yoga. The important thing here is that all doorways into yoga are good. ***Yoga does not care what brings us to yoga. Yoga welcomes all with open arms!*** Any and all reasons, or combination of reasons, for taking up the practice of yoga are good. Whatever our reason is, yoga is big enough to take it. And there is no hierarchy in yoga; there are no deep or superficial motivations. Or put another way: when we practice yoga then our own reasons for practicing are - and can only ever be - the only valid reasons for us. The key point here is that our motivation comes from the inside because when we do not own our motivations then yoga, as a system for empowerment, is just not going to fly.

Which bring us on to the first thing that yoga does care about: yoga cares that we practice. ***Yoga cares that we practice because it is through our practice that yoga reveals its power and beauty to us.*** This power and beauty brings us, whatever our motivation for practicing, time and time again to a point of personal transformation. To realise that transformation, for that opportunity for change to become real, we have to practice and we have to practice regularly. So yoga cares that we commit to a regular practice, and that we each take responsibility or ownership for the work and play that a regular practice brings.

When we step through our doorway into yoga we see many forms of practice. When we think of yoga today the image that will first come to most of us will be the mat-based yoga of the modern yoga class. These classes are typically comprised of sequences of yoga postures, often called Asana, with attention to breathing, often called Pranayama, and meditation. This attention to breathing and meditation is either integrated within the practice of Asana or thrown in at the beginning or end of class for good measure. Today in the West there are many forms of mat-based yoga, all with their own focuses and techniques - the things that make each form distinctive. The creation of a yoga brand around the physical practices is big business in today's yoga industry.

When we look a little deeper we will also see those practicing other forms of yoga. We see the serene calm of the meditators on their cushions and the blissed out faces of the Hare Krishnas as they chant and dance through the city streets. We see those who work tirelessly in all walks of life without any expectation of reward. Again the important thing here is this: *yoga does not care what form our practice takes.* What is important is that, just like our motivations, whatever form our practice takes it is also our doorway to yoga.

Which brings us on to the second thing that yoga cares about: the attitude that we bring to our practice. *And when it comes to attitude yoga cares that we practice with diligence, that we surrender to what our practice brings, and that we use our intelligence.* We will be going into this in a lot more detail throughout the book. As we will see, attitude is the foundation of our yoga practice on our mats and attitude is central to taking our yoga off our mat and into our world. For now this means first and foremost that we let go of our motivations when we roll out our mats. Very simply this is because yoga necessitates working and playing with where we are here and now. Holding on to our motivations is going to mess with our focus on the practice. It is going to mess with our surrender to whatever the practice brings. It is going to mess with our ability to see what is.

What we all share. What we share is that we all come to yoga through our own doorway. We all have our own motivations to practice, and our practice takes many different forms. When we practice regularly there are three more things we all share, three things we all have in common.

The first thing we share is that our yoga works! Our yoga works for each of us in its own way. Whatever the motivation we hold when we first unwrap the box of yoga, odds on our yoga does what it says on the box. It works whether we frame our yoga as a practice for mitigating the effects of stress, as a practice for growing mindfulness, as a practice for building strength, or in any other way. This is the hook that keeps us returning to the practice again and again. And when we let go of our motivation when we practice - or in the words of the yogis of old, we let go of our attachment to the fruits of our actions[1] - then we will bear fruit! Fruit both in terms of our initial motivations, and the fruit yoga throws up along the way. Which brings us on to the second thing we share.

The second thing we share is that yoga wakes us up. Our practice wakes us up in a simple yet very real way. Through practice our perspective on our selves, and the world around us, starts to shift a little. Yoga shifts our attention to things we had taken for granted. Our practice brings things out of the shadows and into the light. We start to see the patterns we have become entangled in and the beliefs about our selves that lie behind these patterns. By bringing these into the light they loose their grip on us. This is therefore a waking up that moves us towards wholeness, towards balance. We move towards our natural state, our source of inner peace and joy, and our source of deeper purpose and original power. Which brings us to the third thing we share.

Yoga wakes us up in a way that is the more that we all want. Wherever we are and whatever course our lives take we all want two things out of life: to feel that we live a meaningful life and to be happy. Our yoga wakes us up to the pursuit of deep happiness; this is the happiness that flows when we grow our connection with our source of freedom and peace, of joy and love. This same source gifts us strength, purpose and creativity, and fills our life with meaning. This is the happiness that flows when we connect with our heart's desire. We share in that we all want to learn how to use the tools of yoga to support us in growing this connection.

Grow awareness! Awareness is the first prop of radically simple yoga. When we start to bring awareness into our yoga practice then we begin to make our yoga real. It is through growing our awareness that we begin to move to own our tipping point. A point where we can effectuate real change in our lives, a point where we are invited to move into the unknown to create something new.

Growing our awareness starts with slowing down. It starts with stopping to reflect before we dance to the tune dictated by our automatic pilot. Because we all have an automatic pilot: one that filters everything according to our likes and dislikes, our beliefs about what is good and what is bad. This automatic pilot operates below the radar, out of sight, and drives and locks us into the patterns we find our selves entangled in. So as we grow our awareness we stop to examine situations from different perspectives. We grow our ability to respond rather than react, and to take responsibility for that response.

When we practice responding from awareness we develop the integration between what we may think of as different parts of our selves. We grow our ability to respond from a place of greater wholeness as the alignment between our thinking, feeling and doing grows. We become more grounded and act from a greater sense of connection inside, connection with our inner source of purpose, joy and peace. The prop of awareness both grows this connection in itself and is the foundation for using all the tools of yoga - such as Asana, Pranayama and meditation - for growing connection.

Awareness is a doorway into depth. It is not the only doorway, and we all come to several doorways as we practice yoga. It is however, a particularly powerful doorway and one that we can all walk through. One we can walk through now because as conscious individuals we all have the capacity to be aware. And as we move into depth through awareness we grow our realisation that the awareness that we have as conscious individuals is a mystery. In other words: the one that is aware is not our true self. The practices of yoga take us down a rabbit hole that is much deeper and much more mysterious than that. Think of awareness as much more akin to a yoga prop. Just like a block. Or better a book used as a block. A book we tear the pages out of as we go along until there is no book there.

Yoga Made Radically Simple

Maps and territories. As our yoga starts to wake us up one consequence is that we begin to see that we have stepped through a doorway into something a lot bigger and a lot more mysterious that we originally thought. And when we move into something big and mysterious it can be useful to have a map: maps help us get our bearings and focus our attention. The sort of map we will be using in this book is called a framework. A framework is a tool that we use to simplify, structure, and communicate reality. Or in other words, a framework is something we can get our heads around. And a good framework is something that supports us as we explore the new and mysterious, it is useful in that respect.

Any traveller who has wandered around a new city with a map in their hand can tell us that the map is not the city. So as we go on our travels through yoga the most important thing to hold in mind about our frameworks is this: *our frameworks are not our reality; they are abstractions, models or metaphors.* This is something the ancients recognised and verbalised in the texts of old, and perhaps most succinctly in the opening line of the Tao Te Ching: *"the Tao called Tao is not Tao."*[2] We will look at the idea of a framework in a bit more detail later on in this section, and return to the mysterious statement on the Tao in Chapter Six.

For the frameworks we will be using to explore yoga in a radically simple way we will be turning to philosophy in general and to yoga philosophy in particular. For the rest of this section we will focus on two things. We will look first at what all philosophical systems have in common. This is our first simple framework and is made up of what we'll call the three big questions. Secondly we will look at what yoga philosophy has to say about these three big questions.

Three questions. Philosophy can at times seem abstract and utterly irrelevant. That is because we have made it that way; we have made it complicated. We have turned it into a head game played inside a high-walled garden that only the initiated are enabled to participate in. So it is time to get radical, time to go back to the roots of philosophy - because that is what radical means. It is time to dig into the simple and powerful core of philosophy.

Odds on you know what that simple core of philosophy is; only you may not know that you know. Because when we ask people what philosophy is then nine times out of ten they will come up with something like: philosophy is thinking about stuff. And that, in a nutshell, is all it is. Philosophy is thinking about stuff, in particular the big questions in life. Philosophy is thinking about the heavy stuff, and thinking about that heavy stuff in a particular way. Philosophers, and that includes all of us, use the tools of reductionism and of synthesis. When we philosophise we dive into the details of a situation - we break things down into parts and explore each part and the relationship between those parts. This is the reductionist part. Then we come back up out of the details to develop frameworks - models - of how these parts all hang together or not. We develop abstractions of reality, and in doing so simplify reality, to help us get some sort of grip on our lives and our world. This is the synthesising part. And when it comes to reductionism all philosophical traditions, both those of the East and those of the West, break down into three main parts or branches.

These three branches deal with three big questions. *The first question is the 'what is this world I find myself in' question. Or simply 'where am I?'* This is a question about the nature of reality. This branch of philosophy is known as metaphysics. The second branch of philosophy is known as epistemology and it deals with the nature and scope of knowledge. *Epistemology deals with questions about what can we know about anything, and in particular* the question: *'who am I?'* The third branch of philosophy deals with what is the right or best way to live. This branch is known as ethics. *This is essentially the 'how am I going to spend my time here' question. Or simply 'what to do?'* These three questions are shown in the illustration below.

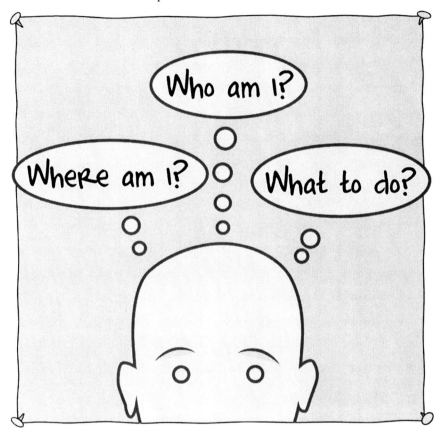

Just like all other philosophical systems, the ancient yoga texts essentially focus on these three questions. However the approaches followed, and the insights communicated, in yoga philosophy are very different to the philosophies of the West that most of us have been brought up with. So let's look at what yoga philosophy has to say about the three big questions and at how yoga philosophy differs from the philosophy of the West.

The big idea of yoga metaphysics is the idea of connection, that we are all one. It is an idea that is found at the core of the most ancient texts of the yogic tradition, the Vedas, and it is the idea that permeates the two most revered texts used in yoga today: the Yoga Sutras of Patanjali and the Bhagavad Gita. This idea of oneness, or wholeness, is the heart of yoga. Oneness as the heart of yoga does not mean that Yoga Philosophy does not use the method of reductionism, the method of breaking things down into parts. We will get to that when we look at the second question. But it is this way round: wholeness is the basis and reduction is a method or a tool. In contrast Western philosophy, and in particular the Western scientific method of much of the last few centuries, has reductionism both as method and as its basis. When it comes to metaphysics in the context of radically simple yoga there is not really anything more to say. The reason for this will become clear when we examine yoga's approach to the second question.

So now let us turn to epistemology, to the question of what we can know about anything, and in particular what we can know about the nature of self. If we take only one thing away from this chapter this is the most important: *yoga in essence is an experiential philosophy.* Experiential means that it is by being and doing that we gain wisdom. Again this contrasts with many strands in Western philosophy that tend towards contemplation. This is why yoga, and yoga teachers everywhere, put so much emphasis on practice: yoga is about commitment to practice rather than to belief. Yoga is non-dogmatic: to practice yoga we do not have to buy into any belief.

The piece above on metaphysics and connection was kept short because yoga basically says: *The cumulative experience of yogis down through the ages is one of connection, that we are all one. We call this the fundamental truth of unity. And don't just take our word for it. Explore it in your own experience, in your own being, through your own practice. It is the wisdom you gain from your personal experience in practice that matters. Go practice, and go manifest the wisdom you gain from your practice when you go out into your world.*

The historians of yoga - and the defenders of certain traditions in yoga - can and will engage in endless debate about the exact origins and development of yoga. However there is one thing that is certain and it is this: the yogis of old did practice. And the wisdom they gained from their experiences they synthesised into a wide variety of frameworks and practices. They developed frameworks to structure and communicate the reality they experienced, and they developed practices for us to work and play with as we go about our own explorations of this reality. Together these frameworks and practices form systems of yoga. Systems that over time the yogis refined, further developed and handed down.

We become familiar with the practices in the modern yoga class environment, practices such as Asana, Pranayama, and meditation. Indeed the role of the modern yoga teacher is most widely interpreted as, and often limited to, instructing students in the technical use of these practices. In contrast this book does not focus on the techniques of practice, but looks at a number of key frameworks distilled from yoga philosophy. It explores in particular how the frameworks and practices mesh together and how to apply these frameworks to empower the practices of yoga on and off our mats. To get us started we will take a closer look at what a framework is and we are going to do this by looking at a couple of examples from Western science.

A framework's value lies in its usefulness! The framework approach is analogous to how mainstream modern science works. So, for example, for a long time physicists took the perspective that an electron can be considered to be a little particle. This was how they slotted the electron into their framework of all matter being categorized as either particles or waves. And the electron as a particle had and has its uses: it can help scientists for example get a grip on how molecules of different elements bond together. Which in turn helps scientists make all kinds of stuff.

However, when scientists started experimenting with how electrons behave under differing conditions they discovered this framework to be incomplete. Yes, at times the electron still seemed to act as a particle; but change the conditions a little and the electron then seemed to act like a wave. These experiments birthed whole new disciplines of physics and for the scientists working in these areas the framework for categorizing electrons as particles or waves is inadequate. For these scientists an electron is much more like a vague blur: a vague blur that has the potential to act both like a particle and like a wave.

There are two important things to note here. Firstly, that the electron, to the early 20th century physicists who were doing these experiments, was what the platypus was to the early zoologists. The platypus is an egg-laying animal that suckles its young, an animal that when discovered by early western zoologists was thought to be a fraud. It did not fit neatly into the framework of mammals and reptiles that the zoologists of the time used to categorize animals. But the platypus was real and it was doing its thing without a care in the world about the zoologist's framework. Likewise the electron did not fit into the scientists' framework of particles and waves. *The point here is that the framework is not the reality.*

The second thing to note is that the ideas of an electron as a particle, as a wave, and as a vague blur all have their uses. For some scientists the particle concept works, for others the wave, and for yet others the concept of a vague blur works better. It depends on what the scientist is looking at, what they are doing. It depends on their perspective. *The point here is that what makes a framework useful is that it works for us from a certain perspective.* The same holds up for the frameworks the yogis developed. *Yoga places the wisdom we get from personal experience through practice first and foremost and offers us frameworks to structure and explore that experience.* The frameworks are maps that we may find useful depending on where we are.

They are not reality and they are not truth. And many of the frameworks the yogis developed are epistemological frameworks: they help us explore the nature of self. We will examine a very simple yet powerful framework for exploring self, and for cultivating our inner attitude to our yoga practice, in the light of these insights into frameworks in the next chapter. But we first need to have a look at yoga's take on that third big philosophical question: what is the right way to live?

A question of ethics? This is where it seems to get a little bit confusing. *It gets confusing because the different traditions that yoga has given rise to have very different approaches to ethics.* On the one hand we have traditions that say: here is an ethical or moral code, start with this and make it the foundation of your practice and your life. Many interpretations of the Ashtanga method given in the Yoga Sutras fall into this category. On the other hand we have traditions that effectively say: focus on sorting out the physical and energetic body, and the mind and ethics will take care of themselves. Hatha Yoga and the Tantra movement fall into this category. To add to the confusion we also have everything in between.

Aside from recognising that different approaches will appeal to different personality types, and each of us as individuals, the main reason for these differences would seem to be that yoga, down through the ages, has become intertwined with other movements. The Hindu religion and the Buddhist tradition in particular have been strong influences. These movements, like yoga, have emerged from the soup of those before them. The influence of this interweaving of movements is evident in both the Bhagavad Gita and the Yoga Sutras of Patanjali. The Bhagavad Gita is steeped in, and is placed within, Hindu mythology. Both Hindu and Buddhist philosophy can be found reflected in parts of the Yoga Sutras.

When, in times gone by, the practitioners of yoga solidified what they found useful into a tradition they often also incorporated ethics. They condensed right ways of living into frameworks of ethics. These codes of ethics form an important foundation for many traditions: they play a role in how the tradition defines itself, and differentiates itself from other traditions. They support the tradition in meeting its primary function of offering structure and sanctuary. And this structure and sanctuary provides real value for many of us. The value of usefulness when we are starting out or when we feel lost, and the value that comes from community. The traditions that place less or little emphasis on frameworks of ethics generally choose to focus on other methods for offering the value of structure and sanctuary.

Wherever our position when it comes to ethics and yoga there are two things to keep in mind. The first thing is this: *a code of ethics in and of itself is empty - it is dead, static.* Whenever we choose to work with a code of ethics, and whatever the prescriptions of that code, we each have to fill it with our own actions to bring it to life in our worlds. Or in other words, the code becomes alive when we are confronted with how to act in the world. The code becomes alive when we face and resolve for our selves the tensions inherent within the gap between the code and all the small and large decisions we make and actions we take. *Our ethics are dynamic when we act in the here and now.*

When we take the perspective that yoga is a system for empowerment the second thing to keep in mind is this: *as we grow awareness and we grow our pool of experiential wisdom the more we can act from this knowledge. We can assume more self-responsibility and act in greater alignment with who we are.* Or in the language of yoga: the more we act from spirit. Frameworks of ethics, like all the frameworks in yoga, can help us on our way by helping us develop our ability to live from spirit. And like all the frameworks in yoga, at some point we move beyond the framework. We move beyond the model and into reality as it unfolds. Otherwise we run the very real risk that the framework, rather than being something that supports us, becomes a hardened veil that keeps us from spirit. And by moving beyond the framework we reclaim the birthright of agency. As we reclaim our agency, we self-realise, we grow our responsibility, our ability to respond unrestricted by method, frameworks and codes.

In summary, when we look at yoga through the lens of philosophy then there are three blocks to yoga: metaphysics, epistemology and ethics. These three blocks address the questions of *'where am I?'*, *'who am I?'*, and *'what to do?'* And down through the ages the different traditions of yoga have given a differing emphasis, and at times differing interpretations, to these three blocks. Traditions, as products of their times, have used these three blocks in specific ways as one of the mechanisms to define the tradition, to set the boundary of what is in and what is out.

Ultimately however, when we practice yoga in a way that is radical - that is aligned with the roots of yoga as a system for empowerment through liberation - then we take the second block as leading. This brings with it a perspective and way of practice that is very simple: it is our quest for self-knowledge that is the foundation of our yoga. *A quest that is experiential in nature and implies that we give the wisdom from our personal experience primacy over adopted ideas.* We give primacy to this wisdom over ideas from outside, over ideas about the nature of reality or the right way to live.

The magic and beauty of yoga is that when we start with the second block then over time the three blocks become one block. It is our own experience that beats the heart of our yoga and reveals our wholeness. It is our knowledge of self that stems from our own experience that informs our worldview and our actions. And this informing forges and strengthens the bond between the three blocks so that over time they become intimately interconnected, they become one, as shown in the illustration below. The danger when we give priority to the first or the third block is that we get stranded in dogma and the three blocks remain three blocks. We hang on to ideas, or struggle to act in ways that are either not grounded or not aligned with the knowledge of self that stems from practice.

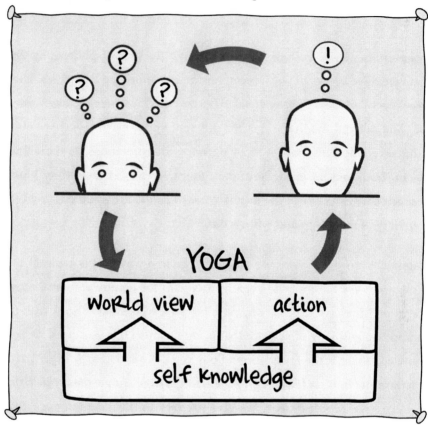

This is the approach that many of the ancients in the West also embraced. Aristotle is claimed to have said: *"knowing your self is the beginning of all wisdom"*[3]. So, using the terminology of Aristotle, yoga provides us with frameworks and tools that will support us in knowing our selves. To embark on the quest for knowledge of self through direct experience and with awareness is yoga made real in action.

Inner Prop: Grow Awareness

The Prop: Growing our awareness means disentangling the part of us that is immersed in experience from the part that can step back and observe. When we grow our awareness we grow our ability to take the perspective of what has been called witnessing consciousness. We take a perspective where we shift our attention away from its habitual captivation by feedback from our bodies and our immediate environment. We shift our attention away from its captivation by clock time and the stories running though our heads. Away from the pulls from family, friends and colleagues around us, from the demands of our daily lives, and from all the non-stop prompting we receive through the media and other cultural mechanisms.

Developing awareness is the first essential skill in making our yoga real. It is through awareness that we grow our ability to see - and be with - things as they are. Training our awareness empowers us by facilitating growth in those characteristics that we cannot train directly such as wisdom and compassion. And training our awareness shifts us from drama trip to dharma trip: it empowers us by shifting us away from characteristics that are holding back our growth, such as resistance to what is and playing victim. And training our awareness empowers us by facilitating growth in our self-response ability, our ability to respond rather than react to stimuli. It is awareness, our witnessing consciousness, which guides our learning and growth.

The first and most important strategy for growing our awareness is to slow down. We slow down in a specific way, we slow down to tune in with our selves, and in a way that creates and lengthens the space between stimulus and response. And this is the space in which that connection to the source inside is found. So as we slow down we create the opportunity to engage from awareness with the present moment as it unfolds rather than reacting with the knee-jerk directions from our automatic pilot. And as we slow down in this way one of the most direct and noticeable effects is that we become happier. We become happier from the inside out. *Now, whilst slowing down does not necessarily mean doing less, a good rule of thumb when starting out is: slow down in any way we can.*

The Prop of Awareness on our Mats: **Our mat-based yoga is a practice of awareness rather than Asana.** One of growing our ability to take perspective rather than do posture. And when we practice yoga on our mats we observe not just with our minds. We observe with our hearts, with our physical body, and we observe energetically. We use the executive function of mind, our ability to direct the attention of our awareness, to bring the intelligence of our full being into the light. Mind is the hand that guides the torchlight of awareness to where the intelligence of our being is asking to be seen. And as we grow our awareness we focus on what is happening in each posture, in each moment, rather than our reaction to it.

Whatever form our mat-based yoga takes the key element is that it is breath-led practice. This is the case whether we are moving or are in stillness. So a good place to start slowing down - and by slowing down to disentangle our awareness - is in our relationship to breath. We focus our attention on the breath and what we find is that what we focus on grows. Through bringing our awareness to the breath we give more space to breath. Or in other words breath deepens, with deepening comes length, and with length comes slowing down. It really is that simple.

So when we roll out our mats we slow down and bring our attention to the breath. And when we move we move with the breath, we move with the inhale and with the exhale. And whilst keeping our attention on the breath, we expand our attention to cover the movement of the physical body. We move with awareness and move with intention. And when we are still we bring our attention to the breath so that our awareness of our physical body is contained within the awareness of the movement of breath.

The Prop of Awareness in our Worlds: It is all too easy to limit growing our awareness to our allocated practice times: those times when we sit down to meditate or when we roll out our mats in yoga class. Other times we are too busy with stuff to do and people to see. We may forget, or tell our selves that we don't have time for the work and play of growing our awareness. We may hold an unconscious belief that it is more efficient to resort to habit. Yet it is outside of our practice times that the real opportunities for transformation present themselves. Awareness only becomes real when we change our whole being in some way - that's what we mean by realisation - we take it out of the realm of thought and intention and into our being.

A good place to start is to bring mindfulness to everyday tasks - tasks such as washing the dishes or brushing our teeth. Tasks we often carry out alone without too much distraction outside. And when we carry out these tasks we slow down inside and we practice taking the perspective of the one observing the one carrying out the task. We observe our selves washing the dishes or brushing our teeth. We observe the breath and we observe the tension that may be present in our physical body. We observe and through observing we create space. And we take this perspective again and again.

And then we grow our awareness in our interactions with others, in our relationships. Again we slow down inside and we practice taking the perspective of the one observing the one interacting. We notice our reactions and we grow space between the input from the other - verbal, attitude and body language, energy - and our reaction. In doing so we grow our ability to respond rather than react. And we play - and this is the real fun part - with shifting our responses in our interactions and relationships.

2. What's Going Down?

We are all intimately, and ultimately, mysteriously connected. This is the message of the ancient yoga of East and the modern science of the West. Yoga is the art of living within and from this mystery. Where there is mystery, curiosity is key.

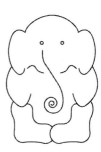

Our Big Shift

Old story, new story: We are living in very exciting times, they are changing and uncertain times. We are living in times characterised by a recognition that the story that has dominated our worldview for hundreds, if not thousands, of years is no longer working. So we are starting to write a new story, and it is a story that has very deep roots: roots that run deep into the fertile ground of that which connects all of us. It is these roots that empower us to acknowledge and take responsibility for the part we all are playing in the new story. They empower us as individuals and empower us as part of the greater whole: they empower us as actors in the story and together as the author. In short, we are living through what has been called a Consciousness Shift. Or to use the term coined by the eco-philosopher Joanna Macy: The Great Turning[4] - because this touches everything. And whatever we call it and wherever we are, it is happening here and it is happening now.

The old story is a story of separation. It is a story of each of us as individuals separate from all others around us, a story of humans as a species separate from the world we live in. It is a story in which we stand apart and above the web of life, and apart and below the realm of spirit. *A story in which we first reject the completeness of the world we find our selves in. And then we succumb to the temptation to lord it over, or play God, in our little material kingdom.* It is a story that we have built on down time, one that has solidified into the systems and behaviours that colour our worldview. It is a story that has brought us real benefits in many areas and one that has brought us just as many illusions of progress.

These illusions of progress are losing their shine. *There is a growing recognition that we are trashing our planet, neglecting and destroying our communities, and losing our selves in the process.* We are waking up to the fact that many of the systems and behaviours that we have constructed around, and that underlie the continuation of, the old story are ultimately destructive. What is important here is that we are all coming to this recognition from our own experience and with our own perspective. As a whole this recognition is wide-ranging, it touches all parts of the old story. It is a recognition that some of us may just be waking up to and one that has been with others for a long time.

For some of us this recognition is rooted in our concerns around our systems of production and consumption: systems that are ravaging our planet, destroying our home, in their relentless quest for more. For others this comes from looking at our money and financial systems. These are systems that have morphed from money as simple currency - from something that flowed and allowed us to share the fruits of our labour and fulfil our basic needs - into highly opaque and complex systems which function to enforce material wealth extraction. Systems that serve the feeding frenzy of the few and that are driving ever more extreme inequality into our community. Or our concerns and recognition may be arising elsewhere - in our food, education or health services systems, anywhere. We are coming from all angles; we are coming from wherever we are.

Whatever our perspective, many of us have two things in common when we look at the old story. Firstly, we recognise that our existing agency structures are unable to address our concerns: agency structures such as our governments of elected and unelected officials and the wide range of commercial entities to which we have delegated responsibility for many areas of our lives. These structures are unable to right the ship. In fact they are more than unable - they cannot be able. *They are dysfunctional and no longer fit for purpose. Simply because they are defined by, and operate within, the boundaries set by the old story.* In a very real sense the only questions of importance become what are going to be the central building blocks of the new story, how are we going to put these blocks together and how the transition from old to new will pan out?

The second thing many of us have in common is that the old story is a story in which we increasingly struggle to find fulfilment and meaning. Somewhere inside of us knows that something very essential has been left out. *Somewhere that knows that buying into this story binds us to a treadmill of frustration in a material wasteland bereft of spirit.* With this we know that spirit - not in any vague sense but spirit as the essence of that which connects us - will be a central building block of the new story.

With this widespread recognition we are starting to move beyond the old story. For many today the statements made in the paragraphs above are not, or no longer, radical or even controversial. This is, in and of itself, a massive step forward and a key motivator for moving forward to create the new. And we are moving forward - the green shoots of the new are everywhere. Whether we look locally or globally, to whatever area of life we turn our gaze, there are people working on the building blocks of a new story. This moving forward develops with stops and starts, with small successes and with failures from which we learn. There are green shoots that have roots that run shallow, and roots that run very deep: that go deep into the heart of the new story, deep into the heart of connection and deep into the heart of yoga.

Before we get into the new story and how yoga plays a part in it, let's dissect the old story a little more. *Because the old story of separation is also a story of inadequacy; when we separate we become incomplete, something is missing.* This is the separation that Descartes famously defined as the seen and unseen, and who gave the seen to the scientists, and the unseen to the church. This separation was an elegant solution to the challenges of the times and effectively formalised - or rubber-stamped - ideas that had been around for a long time. It was a solution that worked out well for a while: at the very least it allowed the scientists to pursue their thing without fear of death on account of heresy.

We did not stop there. *Inadequacy was quickly followed by disempowerment.* The seen became mechanical and we became little cogs in a machine. As cogs we were given something to do and instructions on how to do it, both in a way that was deemed efficient from the perspective of the material; this worked well from the perspective of the machine. These ideas were again rubber-stamped by a couple of scientists - Adam Smith and Frederick Taylor. And these ideas brought with them systems of hierarchy and the belief that we as individuals - as cogs in the machine - were by definition replaceable. These systems, to which we designated our agency, succumbed us and we succumbed to them.

When we frame the old story in terms of Gods then Separation plays the part of Deity-in-Chief, with the lieutenants of Inadequacy and Disempowerment taking place to the left and to the right. Our high priests of reductionism and efficiency closely guard the temples of these deities. These are deities we created, who have always been lifeless, and now is the time to bury them for good. In short it is time for a new story, which of course is also a very old story: the story of connection.

Yoga feeds the deep roots of the story of connection. To understand this we are going to take a short walk through the Bhagavad Gita. The Bhagavad Gita is one of the core texts of yoga and widely considered to be one of the greatest spiritual texts humanity has ever produced. It is a text that has just as much relevance today as when it was written. In essence it is a text that recounts a conversation between the warrior Arjuna and his charioteer. This conversation takes place on a battlefield and is set within the larger mythological tale of the Mahabharata[5].

The Mahabharata is a long convoluted story with countless twists and turns. It is one of India's epic stories and centres around two sets of brothers - the Pandava and Kaurava - who also happen to be cousins. It is a tale full of symbolism: the king who absconds from his throne to retreat into the forest; his blind brother who takes his place, guards the throne, who waivers and changes his mind and action; princes who gamble with their wives at stake; a god who takes on human form and serves a warrior. Although it is far from clear-cut, with falls from grace on both sides, on balance it is the Pandava who represent the benevolent force - an upward evolutionary force.

The conversation laid out in the Bhagavad Gita takes place as the two sets of brothers, once childhood playmates, find themselves facing each other on a battlefield in a dispute over the right to the throne. Arjuna - one of the Pandava brothers - on seeing his family, friends and teachers facing him from across the battlefield hits a wall of indecision. He loses the plot, which is to say he deviates from the warrior script, and sits down to ask his charioteer what he should do. His charioteer is Lord Krishna, divinity incarnate and symbol for oneness, the whole big connected whatever-you-want-to-call-it. By any measure Krishna is a pretty good ally to have commanding your horses as you prepare for battle. Rather than directly telling Arjuna what to do, Krishna instructs him in yoga. *And in essence Krishna tells Arjuna just three things: three things that capture the blessing and burden of yoga.*

The first thing Krishna tells Arjuna: *'Wake up! You are not who you think you are. We are all connected, with each other, with everything. We all have the spark of divinity in us, and the spark of divinity in me is the spark of divinity in you. We all are One.'* Clear and simple, and so on to the second thing: *'Whilst we are all One, you are also here and now, in space and in time. And there is no place to hide! Exercise your agency. You are the One, and also the one that acts and produces effect in this world. You have spent your lifetime exploring and building your talents, now act accordingly.'*

These first two things that Krishna tells Arjuna are what are often thought of - and brought to us - as two of the paths of yoga: the path of knowledge, known as Jnana yoga, and the path of action, known as Karma yoga. These two things may appear to contain a contradiction: all is One, and you are an individual. They are traditionally, and we will dig a little deeper into tradition in just a moment, brought as a choice: a choice between paths - between Karma yoga, Jnana yoga - and the path often distilled from the third thing that Krishna tells Arjuna, the path of Devotion or Bhakti yoga. *Happily the essence of the third thing that Krishna tells Arjuna both resolves the apparent contradiction and shatters the illusion of a choice between paths.*

Because the third thing that Krishna tells Arjuna is: *'Love me! Dedicate all to me - to the One. Act in the knowledge that you are within the oneness and act in the knowledge that what you do matters. Intention from this knowledge realised in action is love.'* *Or in short - act in the good of the whole.* These three things not only contain the essence of Krishna's instruction in yoga, they also speak to the three big philosophical questions we touched on in Chapter One. Then Krishna passes the ball to Arjuna and says: *'you choose'*. And Arjuna, after hearing all Krishna has to say, picks up his weapons and takes to the battlefield.

We are going to dig a whole lot deeper into the Bhagavad Gita in Chapter Five. In particular we will look at the Bhagavad Gita as myth or metaphor and at the warrior archetype. For now let's keep to Krishna's message in the context of the new story. *And the radically simple message of the Bhagavad Gita is one of holistic agency.* It is a message of unity and from unity empowerment, one of fulfilling our purpose in the service of all. *This message contains a refuge, the blessing of yoga, and a responsibility, the burden of yoga.* Or it could be that the refuge is the burden, and the responsibility the blessing. Or it may be both or neither.

Krishna's message is one that strikes to the heart of the new story. Because although we do not know how the new story will manifest there are a few things we do know. Firstly, we know that the new story will be told from an exploration of connection - or what the yogis of old called the fundamental truth of unity. Secondly, we know that the new story will be written from the bottom up - that we each have a part to play. It will be written from the bottom up because that is an undisputable implication of reclaiming our agency. And thirdly, we know that the deeper the realisation of connection the more resilient the new story will be - and resilient it will need to be. Just like in Arjuna's times there is a war going on: a war between the upward force of the new story and the downward force of the old.

Krishna's message is one that feeds the new story in a way that is both deeply spiritual and personally practical. It is spiritual because by acting for the good of the whole we resolve the apparent contradiction between the One and one. And practically it is a message that speaks to all of us wherever we are. Because we are all here and we are all doing some sort of something or other. In essence Krishna's message is not a choice of paths - the path of Jnana, Karma or Bhakti yoga. The choice is much more simple and radical than that. The choice is one of grounding within, and taking action from, spirit: the choice of what persona do we manifest. And just like in the tale of the Mahabharata our personal stories are convoluted, they are complex. The choice, however convoluted our story, is between the upward thrust of evolution - towards light - and a downward thrust towards darkness. The choice, that through yoga becomes an exploratory obligation, of manifesting love through action.

The shift in story necessitates a shift in our yoga. Whatever its history, mat-based yoga really took off when yoga came to the West. This success has been largely driven by two interplaying factors. *Firstly there was, and is, a great need for yoga as a healing practice in the West.* And yoga practice supports us in repairing the damage inside that we incur from living within the old story. Yoga supports us in growing wholeness inside and grows our connection to spirit in whatever form we frame it. This is a need for yoga that simply - in a very down to earth and yet powerful way - supports us in feeling better about our selves. As a result yoga in the West has largely been co-opted within the well-being sector: *yoga for health and relaxation is the dominant new yoga tradition we have built in the West.*

The second factor behind the success of yoga in the West has been the ability of the West to turn yoga into a commodity. This should come as no surprise as turning stuff into commodities is an integral part of the old story. It is a skill we in the West have developed and honed to perfection as we have fine-tuned the old story. *And so we have the modern business of yoga built around yoga as commodity.* This is yoga as a thing with a well and externally defined set of attributes that can be bought and sold in the marketplace. We see the manifestation of this commoditisation in the proliferation of yoga brands, the overbearing obsession with method and technique, the pimping of spiritual accessories and the rise of the yoga teacher as celebrity or personality.

To be very clear: there is nothing wrong with either of these two factors. The business of yoga has driven the growth of yoga's reach. Commoditisation has opened the door of yoga to us all and it is by walking through that door that many of us found our way to yoga. And the new tradition of yoga as a well-being practice not only filled a need, it is an essential part of writing a new story. As the ancients knew only too well: healing starts inside. Neither, as anyone who has spent time in India knows, is any of this new. In India they know how to dress up and sell stuff as well as anyone and down through the ages the simple and powerful messages of yoga have been packaged in different metaphors and narratives. How these messages have been brought and taught to us has morphed and adapted to fit the cultural context of the times. They have been surrounded in different rituals. This is how traditions are birthed. And one thing that is certainly true of yoga is that yoga has birthed a lot of traditions.

However traditions are a double-edged sword. This holds both for our new yoga as well-being tradition and the different traditions of yoga down through the ages. The defining characteristic of double-edged swords is that they cut two ways. Cut one-way traditions offer structure and they offer sanctuary, both of which can be good - as in useful - things: in the past, now, and in the future. To offer both they use specific practices, myth and story, rituals and codes. In fact traditions use anything they can get their hands on to capture and package what they think is valuable. And in doing this, traditions create a boundary between what is in and what is out. Which brings us on to the other way the sword of tradition cuts. Because by capturing and packaging experience and learning they create something that is solid and static - a calcified shell that surrounds the beating heart of yoga.

The shift in our yoga that the story of connection necessitates is a shift away from yoga as a commodity. And it is a shift that builds on - and grows hand in hand with - our new tradition of yoga as a well-being practice. It is a shift that expands our attention from yoga as a system for inner healing to one for inner and outer healing. A shift towards yoga as a system for personal empowerment: personal empowerment that is aligned with, and flows from, the essence of Krishna's message to Arjuna. This is a very specific form of empowerment that is aligned with the message that the One is telling itself as the ones who act and produce effect. This message comes from deep within and without our selves and is calling: heal me - come out of hiding and play your part. This is a shift in our yoga that requires nothing new as everything is already perfectly in place. The only thing this shift requires is for each of us to explore - and through exploring - engage in the adventure with the beating heart of yoga.

This adventure starts with coming back to basics and with working from the bottom up. From the bottom up means recognising that above anything yoga is about authentic personal experience, about working and playing with our own experience. Experience that - as outlined in Krishna's message to Arjuna - is characterised both of being individuals and of being part of a whole: of being one and of being in Oneness. And coming back to basics means focusing on the core of the yoga. This is the core that lies beyond the specifics of individual methods, techniques and tools. And it is a core that is universally applicable wherever we are and whatever our individual situations, possibilities and differences. It is this core that we have started to explore in Chapter One and will continue to explore throughout this book. And when we go on an exploration then a good tool to have in our toolbox is curiosity.

Get curious! Curiosity is the second prop of radically simple yoga: it is an essential attitude as we make our yoga real. It is a skill, or prop, we are all gifted; although it may have lost its shine or been misdirected as we go through life. As we saw in Chapter One, one of the things we all have in common as we practice yoga is that yoga wakes us up and one consequence of this waking up is that at some point we realise that we have stepped into something that is larger or different than we had expected when we started off. The same holds true for curiosity. Yoga wakes us up to the realisation that our curiosity is a much broader and deeper skill than we may think it is.

We have been conditioned to believe that curiosity is limited to our thinking. We have been conditioned by the old story of separation to believe that our ability to be curious, and our ability to be aware and intelligent, is defined by what is going on in our heads. Our practice of yoga shifts this. *Through our practice we develop a curiosity that is holistic - we develop our ability to take our awareness deep down into our being.* And as we go down we get curious about our own experience. We become curious about our experience from a position of awareness, from a position that is disentangled and non-violent. Most importantly we get curious about feeling, about sensation unfiltered by mind and story. *This feeling is the intelligence of our being speaking to us. It is the intelligence of the One speaking to us.* And that is a pretty big shift for many of us.

To understand this we have to do a bit of headwork. This is the self-reinforcing virtuous circle of the intelligence of our head and body. Or it is the catch-22 of yoga philosophy depending on our perspective. And the headwork we are going to do is a short exploration of science and yoga. Because if there is one characteristic that stands out in our times it is that of increasing globalisation. We live in a time where West meets East, and East meets West, and with this meeting comes an increasing entanglement of societies and cultures. After all this is how we in the West came to yoga.

At its most fundamental level this is a meeting of worldviews: a meeting of belief systems. The dominant belief system of our times in the West is science. We in the West have all been deeply infused with scientific thinking whether we think of our selves as identifying with science or not. And science, just like yoga, has a lot of mystique around it. So let's lift the veil and take a peek at what's really going down when the science of the West meets that of the yoga of the East. We will look first at the big picture and then we will zoom in on what science and yoga have to say about the mystery of consciousness.

When East Meets West

Same same but different! When the philosophies and practices of the ancient East meet the scientific thinking of the West they may seem like two completely different worlds. At first glance these two thought systems approach the big questions of life from different perspectives. Very simply yoga, and with it Eastern spirituality in general, is holistic. It takes the perspective and builds on the power of what is called the fundamental truth of unity. Western scientific thinking is reductionist. It takes the perspective and builds on the power of breaking things down into little pieces.

When we hear the terms science and yoga this tends to conjure up images of the application of the scientific method to prove or disprove benefits or risks that yoga practice may bring. However when science meets yoga the resulting message is a lot bigger than the statistics of whether certain forms of Asana practice can lead to injury or improve our sex lives. Statistics, that incidentally in many cases have little to do with science, as they do not take into account whether the subjects are actually practicing yoga or just jumping around on a mat[6]. The message is a lot bigger because when we dig a little deeper we see that these two systems have a lot more in common than we often think. We find that although they use a different language they are nudging up towards the same message, both with respect to the big picture of life and also when it comes to our own lives. This is the stuff that is really compelling. It is compelling because it is powerful and concerns each of us, and right now we are going to look at three things.

The first thing that science and yoga agree on is this: *we live in a deeply interconnected world.* It has taken science a while to get there because for a long time the story of science was the story of separation. Separation was central as scientists moved both up and down in scale when considering pieces of reality. Because as our scientific thought system and technological ability have grown one important consequence has been that scientists became able to explore the very small and the very large. They have moved down from molecules, to atoms, to sub-atomic particles, and they have moved up from our planet, to the solar system, to galaxies and entire universes.

It was when physicists moved down into the sub-atomic world that the method of scientific reductionism, and the idea of a world made up of separate objects, ran up against a wall. They ran up against this wall when they were carrying out exactly those experiments we introduced in Chapter One when we looked at electrons as particles or waves in the context of frameworks. What they discovered is that at its deepest level our material reality cannot be divided into individual pieces, i.e. the basic fabric of the universe is inherently indivisible - everything is connected to everything else. So at a very deep level, at the level of the most fundamental stuff - what ever that is - we are all connected to each other. And we are all connected to galaxies far away. Rather than distinct from the world around us, we are deeply entangled with it. We are an intimate part of the whole. This is a key insight of the modern science of quantum physics. *And an insight long proclaimed short and sweet in the yoga tradition: we are all one.*

The second thing that science and yoga agree on is this: *the best metaphor we have for the fabric of our connection is some sort of energy.* In the language of science, the metaphor that science uses, the basic indivisible fabric of everything is a vast ocean of energy. Scientists and commentators look at this ocean from differing perspectives and have given it various names, such as the quantum field, the zero-point field, the unified field, or simply the field. Science maintains that everything, both the intangible and that which we perceive in our material world, arises out of this field of energy. And science maintains that everything, including each of us, at its most fundamental level can be seen as an energy charge or cluster.

The holistic spiritual philosophies of the ancient East use a slightly different metaphor for describing this energy field; it is known as the life force. Gandhi explicitly acknowledged the inherent unknowableness of this energy field when he called it an *'indefinable mysterious power'*[7]. In different traditions of the East, and in the more mystical strands of Western religion, this life force has been given different names. The yogis for example call it Prana, and the Taoists call it Chi. In the Western Christian tradition it is known as the Holy Spirit. Spiritual traditions across the world call it Love. Analogous to the energy charges of science, in the metaphor of the East everything we perceive is a manifestation of this life force. Right now a popular metaphor used by both science and yoga for this ocean of energy or life force is consciousness. This is a word that evokes some form of intelligence for the energy that permeates everything. So when it comes to science and yoga it is so far, so good: we are all connected and we use the idea of energy for the metaphor for that which connects us.

The mystery begins here! **The third thing that science and yoga have in common is that neither science nor yoga can tell us the full story of our relationship with this ocean of energy or life force.** Or in terms of the metaphor of consciousness, neither can tell us what the relationship is between our individual consciousness and the greater consciousness or life force that connects us. For science and yoga, consciousness, and therefore our awareness that just may well be a function of consciousness, is a mystery.

Now this third point is important, very important, so we will look in a bit more detail at how science and yoga approach this mystery. For a long time science basically passed over the whole consciousness thing. It was considered too slippery or intractable and, to put it very crassly, one could not make a scientific career out of studying consciousness. This changed around twenty years ago. A reframing of efforts to understand consciousness by the philosopher David Chalmers known as 'The Hard Problem'[8] coupled with technological developments to allow scientists to delve ever deeper into the human brain has led to a huge amount of work in this area. This work has lead to all sorts of specialist fields in the area of brain science.

Within the scientific community The Hard Problem tends to polarise discussion: debates amongst scientists, and between scientists and philosophers, get heated, anger rises and insults are thrown. This, for outsiders to the technical intricacies, is a sure sign that mystery is present and assumptions are being made. And whilst there are all sorts of opinions out there, it is safe to say that most scientists *appear to believe* that consciousness is a function of brain activity. The new fields of brain science focus - at the most fundamental level - to provide support for this belief. Thus most scientists frame The Hard Problem of consciousness as an endeavour to join the dots between how the measurable activity of our brain gives rise to our experience as conscious individuals. And for many scientists The Hard Problem is hard because they are not sure what sort of answer they are looking for.

For our discussion a key thing to note is that the way most scientists frame The Hard Problem is founded upon, and reinforces, a separation. The very way the question is formulated locks in perspective. Consciousness starts and ends with the brain. This locking in rests on faith: the faith that comes with the opportunity and burden that Descartes gave to science when he formalised a separation between spirit and matter. When we shift to the perspective of connection, and the mysterious energy that connects us, the possibility arises that the hardness in this question comes from the way the question is framed. Rather than having no idea what kind of answer to expect, it may be that science - by locking in perspective - does not know what kind of question to pose.

So when we start to explore our beliefs around separation and connection we are invited to explore to what extent modern brain science, and science in general, will ever succeed in its quest. Will science ever be able to tell the story of our relationship with life force? Or in other words, we are invited to entertain the idea that we - with our conscious minds - cannot tell the full story of consciousness. We are invited to sit up and ask: *is mind attempting to tell the story of consciousness using thought the mind working as an Idiot Box in full flow?* So at this point in time, when East meets West, the idea we are invited to entertain is that the reductionism of science is not a method fit for telling this story.

There is another angle to this invitation, and it involves us taking a side step into the world of mathematics. Mathematics is relevant because mathematics is the language of science. It is a tool that scientists and philosophers use to define things in a very abstract way using numbers and symbols, and to describe the relationships between them. Or in other words, mathematics is a psychological and social construct and it is the mother tongue in the land of separation. And the foundation of mathematics is a branch of mathematics known as logic.

For a long time mathematicians were caught in a quest to show that logic itself was built on solid ground: they wanted to show that the foundations of the language of science were solid. Because for science this would be a good thing - good to know that science is built on hard rock and not on soft sand. This quest was abruptly brought to a halt in the 1930s when the logician Gödel demonstrated that any attempt to build an irrefutably solid basis to logic using logic was doomed to failure. Or in other words: we cannot pull our selves up to the peak of the mountain of knowledge using our own bootstraps. Gödel, incidentally, spent significant portions of his later life hospitalised due to mental instability.

For the vast majority of scientific endeavours the implications of Gödel's work can be put to one side. In addition to the obvious allure of not having to risk going through what Gödel went through, scientists can continue to explore and to make stuff. They make stuff that works well. However when we come to consciousness and mind, the implications would appear to be real. When science is attempting to tell the story of mind, of consciousness, it uses a language of mind that is in itself incomplete. It is a language that is either built on rock or sand, neither or both. We just don't know. *So again, the idea we are invited to entertain is that the reductionism of science will never be able to tell the full story of our relationship with life force.* That in this respect the scientific method is not fit for purpose.

The idea of separation of spirit and matter, and the method of reductionism of science, run deep. They permeate the perspectives that each of us takes a lot of the time, and in many areas of our lives. They go far beyond only being an approach adopted by the professional scientists at their desks and in their laboratories. In a very real way we are all Descartes' children. And the invitation to let go of separation and reductionism goes far beyond a mere intellectual exercise. It is an invitation to absorb and make real in our own being and doing. Happily there are tried and tested personal empowerment systems to support us when we engage with this invitation: systems such as yoga.

Practice Yoga! Another way of looking at the joining the dots question is to entertain the proposition that mainstream Western science may never be able to understand the link between our selves as conscious observers and the greater consciousness all around us. And this is the essence of what the science of yoga discovered long ago. The yogis explored the importance of consciousness in our subjective experience. They explored moving through their subjective experience into a greater consciousness beyond. They loosened themselves from the thought patterns of little mind to move into greater mind. And they discovered that they couldn't give us the answer. *They discovered that consciousness is a mystery. That any attempt to box it in with mind will fall short.*

In the West we have been conditioned to expect answers, to expect explanations. *The message of both science and yoga is as radical as it is simple: beware of consciousness as the new God metaphor.* So it is when we look at consciousness that our story of science and yoga begins to get murky. And as far as you and me are concerned murky is a good thing: murky is where the mystery begins. Murky is where there is space to explore, where it begins to get juicy. In summary when it comes down to the three points we have discussed science and yoga offer complementary rather than competing views. *The bottom line is it is not where or how we get our knowledge that matters. It is what we do with it.*

When it comes to the quest of joining the dots, the approach of yoga is very different to that of Western science. Rather than examining the ocean of energy, the mystery of life force, from the outside yoga invites us to dive into the ocean, to engage directly with life force. The yogis discovered that the joining of these dots is not a story to be told by mind. For the yogi to rise to the quest is to accept the invitation, and obligation of, personal exploration. This is the heart of the yogi's science of the mind, a science that in essence is very different to the modern Western science. As yogis we embark on an experiential process. We embark on a process where we move from our thinking mind - the mind that tells stories and that mandates knowing - into the holistic intelligence of our being. A process that involves growing our ability to listen, and to listen not just through our ears but also in all ways we can. A process that necessitates tapping into the intelligence of the Oneness as it speaks to us.

One way of looking at yoga is that it is a system, a set of tools and processes, for directing this exploration. Although yoga is not the only system for this it is a particularly effective one: because yoga can be personalised to each and every individual. Yoga is also effective because yoga goes deep - yoga has the potential to reach the parts other systems may not. So through yoga we explore what is going down for us. The thoughts we are having, the emotions we are feeling and the actions we are doing. Or when we shift the lens of our exploration, the thought, emotional, and doing patterns that are doing us. So it is time to introduce another framework, a simple and powerful framework to support us in this exploration. We are going to call this framework the philosopher's simple anatomy.

Our belly, head and heart. When we hear the word anatomy we tend to think of bones, muscles, joints and organs. We may think of bodily systems like our respiratory, digestive and circulatory systems. This is the standard fare of human anatomy at school and it is also the bricks and mortar of anatomy teaching for mat-based yoga today. All thorough trainings for yoga teachers include modules on the muscular-skeletal system and on the main organs and physical systems in the body. This is a necessary and good thing. The ability to visualise and understand the connections in our physical body is a key element in personalising the practices of Asana in a way that is both safe and functional for us.

Many forms of mat-based yoga also go further. They include teachings on subtle anatomy; these are the frameworks that yoga has come up with to describe our bodily experience from the perspective of energy. Based on their experience the yogis developed the model of seven energy centres or chakras. They came up with the system of three main, and thousands of other, energy pathways within the body. And they came up with specific practices to purify and open up the energy pathways and centres. Again this is all good and necessary stuff. Expanding our perspective from our physical body and into our energetic experience is at the heart of yoga as a breath-led practice. And as we move deeper it is an essential step in exploring mystery and an intimate part of growing our ability to embrace life.

The philosophers of yoga use a much simpler framework than those of both physical and subtle anatomy. *This framework stems from our collective experience that we are doing, thinking and feeling beings.* And it is a framework that recognises that our power, or energy, for these aspects of our being lie in our belly, head and heart respectively. This framework is shown in the illustration below.

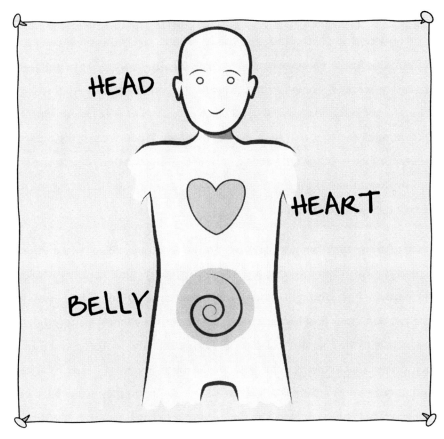

This idea is not one exclusive to yoga. It is common to many systems both in the East and West. In the East this is perhaps most explicit in the Chinese Taoist tradition. The Taoists use a model of the three Dantians[9], meaning centres or literally fields of heaven: the lower, the upper, and the middle Dantian. Analogously around 2,000 years ago in the West Plato postulated that: *"The human soul is composed of three parts - the appetite, the rational, and the spirit."*[10] And religious traditions all around the world are centred on the three pillars of service, mindfulness and gratitude, albeit given different names.

Modern science also has some very useful and powerful messages to tell us in respect to this framework: messages about thought, about the interconnectedness of mind and body, about our power as conscious individuals. These messages are not negated in any way by any limitations of science when it comes to the mystery of consciousness. And when it comes to our belly, head and heart science tells us: **that what we do matters, that thought matters, and how we feel matters.** When we put the mystery of consciousness, or the red herring of who is doing the thinking, to one side for a moment then this is the mandate of empowerment and reclaiming our agency that science gives us.

Science knows that thought plays a central role in our subjective experience of reality. The modern sciences of neurobiology and neuropsychology can explain how thought drives our experience of life. How thought, whether conscious and unconscious, plays out in our emotions through the production of the chemicals of emotion. Emotion, how we feel about things, then drives our behaviour. So thought, through emotion, leads to action. And science knows there is a feedback loop, so action then feeds back into thought. This feedback loop has the potential to catch us up in patterns of thinking, feeling and doing.

Science also knows that our subjective experience plays out at the objective level: that what we experience inside in terms of thought and feeling produces changes that can be measured. What we think and how we feel manifests in our physical bodies, and this impacts our doing and manifests through our connections and into our worlds. Science can show that when we truly learn, learn not just at the cognitive level but grow our ability to behave differently we incorporate this wisdom in our cells. It is by action, and in particular through repetition, that we create new neural nets - hardwired pieces of knowledge - in our brains. This is how we loosen our selves from one pattern and create another.

These three centres - or pillars - are at the core of all forms of yoga practice. They permeate through and through those two yoga texts of old, the Yoga Sutras and the Bhagavad Gita, although the messages in these texts are packaged in different metaphors and narratives. The way they are brought and taught to us may make them appear different - through time the language used has been adapted to fit with differing traditions and cultural conditions. And the two texts present different methods or tools. However when it comes to our belly, head and heart, the yoga of the Yoga Sutras is the yoga of the Bhagavad Gita: at the end of the day it's all one yoga.

The Yoga Sutras and the Bhagavad Gita do place yoga in different contexts. Broadly speaking we can say that the Yoga Sutras focuses more on practices to go inside whilst the Bhagavad Gita focuses more on taking yoga into the world. We will be looking more closely at both these texts in the next few chapters. For now we will simply introduce the practices - or yogas - in these texts in the context of our belly, head and heart. The key elements of each that relate to our simple anatomy. In the Yoga Sutras this is Kriya Yoga, the practices of Tapah, Svadhyaya and Isvara-Pranidhana. These are, in plain English, the practice of dedication to, and purification through, practice, the practice of self-study and the practice of surrender to what is. These three practices are rooted in our bellies, heads and hearts, and whatever outer form our practice of yoga on our mats takes we engage in these three practices. As we have seen earlier, in the Bhagavad Gita these practices are known as Karma yoga, Jnana yoga and Bhakti yoga - the yogas of selfless service, knowledge, and devotion.

We will be returning to this simple framework of belly, head and heart throughout this book because it is a powerful framework. It is powerful because it is a framework we can all relate to and work with on and off our mats. And it is powerful because it is simple: in general the simpler a framework is the more powerful it is. We will also look at moving beyond this framework - reminding our selves that it is just a model.

We are not human doings, human thinkings, or human feelings: we are human beings. We are human beings that from one perspective can be framed as a belly, head and heart, from another as an energy charge, and from yet another as a bag of flesh and bones. When we bring yoga into our lives - on and off our mats - we work and play with our one indivisible being. In a very real way we are aligning and integrating our three power centres of doing, thinking, and feeling. These three power centres are always connected but they just may be a little out of whack. As we grow connection between these centres we grow our ability to fully participate in life from moment to moment. We rise to the ongoing challenge and invitation in each moment to act with love, to perceive through love, and to open our heart to love. And through our yoga we start to undergo a specific sort of transformation. This is a transformation that will manifest in its own way for each of us: transformation inside and outside, on and off our yoga mat. This is a specific sort of transformation that yoga needs right now, and that the world at large needs. This transformation begins with getting curious from awareness and that is yoga made real in action.

Inner Prop: Get Curious

The Prop: Let's get one thing clear up front: curiosity did not kill the cat. Worry and sorrow killed the cat. Whether by intent or by chance the original saying morphed into what we have today. In contrast, in yoga as in life, curiosity is a good quality, and the good thing about curiosity is that it is a trainable skill, a skill we can all develop. An even better thing about curiosity is that it is fun. Curiosity brings play and lightness into our practice and life. It is when we layer curiosity onto awareness that we really start to make our yoga real.

The most effective way to train our curiosity is by asking questions. In yoga we begin with asking questions that stem from that very basic question: *'what is going down here and now?'* We may start with questions that have an answer, questions like: what is colouring my experience right now, what is the function of this Asana for me, how does it feel when I do this differently, what is going on with breath, thought and emotion? And as our practice deepens we start to engage with questions that have no answer: questions where the ongoing exploration is the answer.

When we start asking questions we very literally start to open up our minds: the very act of asking the question brings space into where we had locked down our perspective through making up our mind. So by making space in opening our minds we grow our ability to see things as they are. We loosen our selves from the filters of our perception and develop what the yogis of old called Samadhi, or neutral vision[11]. And seeing things the way they are opens our hearts. Opening our hearts leads to acceptance, to compassion and to love. So when we train our curiosity from awareness we grow our openness to these sorts of qualities: we facilitate the growth of qualities that we cannot train directly. Growing acceptance and compassion leaves less room for worry and sorrow. Which brings us back to the cat.

The Prop of Curiosity on our Mats: **Our mat-based yoga practice is in essence one of unbounded curiosity rather than having answers.** The physical practices of yoga are explicitly designed to awaken our curiosity, and in particular to get us curious about our own experience. We get curious about our physical bodies, the thoughts and emotions that bubble up into our awareness, about our relationship with breath. Applying our curiosity to our framework of belly, head and heart provides a pretty good starting point for developing the sort of curiosity that is going to take us deeper into yoga.

For many of us it is the feedback coming from our physical bodies - from the doing of our belly - and from the voice in our heads that is most manifest when we roll out our mats and practice. With curiosity we start to investigate what is going on in our physical bodies and we develop the ability to feel into where we experience tightness or resistance. We get better at locating sensation within our body, and we learn to distinguish between the flashing red light of pain that says stop, and what some yogis have called sweet pain. This sweet pain is the pain that arises from some part of us asking for attention.

As we get curious about the voice in our head we start to notice what is captivating our attention, what pulls us away from the here and now, and away from our work at hand. We get curious about these distractions, and how they manifest as stories told in our heads, and curious about how we can acknowledge them and yet not become entangled in them. *We start to get curious about our automatic pilot's likes and dislikes. These are the things that are driving our habitual behaviour on and off our mats.*

As we start to look at what is most manifest - at what is both very simple and very real - we connect with our hearts. We explore how we can manifest compassion for our selves in each moment of our practice. We start asking questions of our being to investigate what it means to embrace the challenges of our practice on our mats with an open heart. *And perhaps most importantly of all we start to get curious about our relationship with breath.* Where is breath flowing and where does it feel blocked? Is the breath coming in and out of us deep or shallow, long or short? What happens with mind as breath lengthens and deepens? What happens with the sensation in our physical body when we direct our attention and breath to the places where we feel blocked?

The Prop of Curiosity in our Worlds: Once we have started to cultivate awareness in our worlds then getting curious from that position of awareness flows naturally. When we notice things without being entangled - or invested - in that thing, then the space is there for inquiry. So let's look again at those two situations we introduced with the prop of awareness - everyday tasks and our relationships with others.

Once we bring curiosity from awareness into our everyday tasks and all of our relationships what we will notice is pattern. It may be a pattern of gripping the dishcloth as we wash the dishes, or holding onto the toothbrush for dear life as we brush our teeth. It may be a pattern of resistance to tasks we don't like: a pattern that manifests as a story in our heads, a closing in our heart, a rush to move to the next thing in our doing. And in relationships it may be a pattern of jumping to conclusions about the intention of the other, one of shortness, one of always wanting to please or a craving for recognition. Or it may be something else altogether. Whatever it is, the practice of listening with curiosity with our full being will shed light.

An important thing about such patterns is that they are personal and real. They are real in the sense that they drive our experience of life from moment to moment. And whilst they are personal they are also commonplace. So in all these ways they are very ordinary - there is nothing esoteric or mystical about them. And this matters. To quote two lines from the Tao Te Ching: *"Understanding the ordinary: mind opens. Mind opening leads to compassion."*[12]

3. Exploring Connection Inside

When we practice yoga on our mats we work and play within our breath and with our attitude. We loosen our selves from the patterns we have become entangled in. Our non-violent surrender to what our practice brings liberates and empowers us.

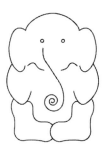

The Yoga of the Yoga Sutras

Heal our selves! The invitation of the Yoga Sutras is to heal our selves, to rediscover our wholeness. *To rediscover our wholeness implies loosening our selves from patterns that reinforce the illusion of separateness.* Because the basic characteristic of patterns is that they impose a structure that brings partition, and we all get entangled in pattern. We become deeply embedded in patterns, both as individuals and collectively. Individually these patterns manifest as our habits and addictions, as the accessories of our persona, as parts of who we believe we are. Collectively these patterns manifest as ways of organising our selves in tribes, communities and societies; they manifest in our cultures, structures and law.

From one perspective we need patterns to go about our lives. In this respect there are patterns that in a very practical way work for us, that is they support our growth, and patterns that don't. From this perspective our yoga practice may function as a tool for recognising patterns for what they are, and for sifting through these patterns. Our practice serves to strengthen healthy patterns that support us in growing our feeling of wholeness, and for weakening unhealthy patterns. However from another perspective identification with any pattern reinforces the illusion of separation. This identification clouds our experience of our wholeness; it limits our being in the here and now. From this perspective our yoga is a dissolving of our identification, or entanglement, with pattern. *This is the yoga of the Yoga Sutras, the yoga of growing connection inside.*

The yoga of loosening our selves from patterns starts with growing our choice of perspective, of seeing patterns for what they are. As we start to grow our sense of wholeness inside this process spills over and dissolves the boundaries between what we thought is inside and what is outside. But before we dig a little deeper into the Yoga Sutras let's introduce another framework. This is a simple map - or model - that sheds some light on how patterns manifest at our individual level and one that will support us when we turn again to the Yoga Sutras. This simple framework characterises patterns by the state we find our selves in: states such as openness or resistance; a state of peace or one of fear; relaxation or stress. These are common everyday states that drive our behaviours and that lock us into habitual patterns of being and of doing. This simple framework is shown below[13].

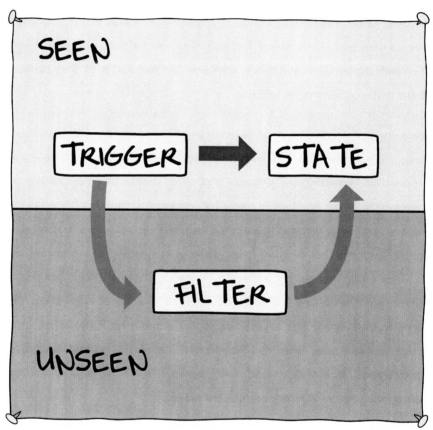

What the framework in this illustration shows us is that we find our selves in a certain state because of our reaction to certain triggers in our worlds. These triggers arise from our internal system - such as feelings of hunger, warmth, cold or tiredness. Or they arise from our interactions with the world around us - typically from our immediate environment and very often from our interactions with others such as family, friends and colleagues. *And the framework shows us that we experience our reactions as automatic.* That is, the trigger arises and before we know it we find our selves in a certain state - this is the thick black arrow in the illustration. Our conscious experience is one of trigger and then state: a state that could be functional but often is pure habit. The well-known example is that of running up against a tiger in the forest where we react with a state of stress. A state that in this example is functional: we are in a life-threatening situation and it primes us for fight or, in all probability the wiser strategy of, flight. However when our stress reaction becomes habitual we find our selves in a state of stress as a reaction to all sorts of non-life-threatening situations. It may be as a reaction to interactions with certain individuals or to the seemingly non-stop demands of our modern lives.

What the illustration also shows us is that our automatic pilot actually functions using a sorting mechanism that we call filters – this is the grey curved arrow in the illustration. *That is our automatic pilot uses filters to process triggers and to determine and drive our reaction into state: the filters function as our lens of perception.* This opens the possibility that it is not - or at least not only - the trigger that drives our state but also how we process this internally. Now most of the time we are unaware of this sorting process - that is why we call it our automatic pilot. So although we are usually aware of the trigger and our state, we are not aware of our filters. Or in other words the trigger and the state are seen, and the filters are unseen.

In essence what this framework is showing us is that when we are entangled in pattern we react in the same way each time we run up against certain triggers. In other words entanglement in pattern dictates that we spend our time dancing to the tune of our automatic pilot. Or framed in the language of the old story of separation - the story of the material world - we are conditioned, and have conditioned our selves, to react mechanically to triggers.

Now let's return to the Yoga Sutras and the yoga of growing connection inside. This focus on growing connection inside explains why the Yoga Sutras are generally considered to present yoga in the monastic tradition. Simply because in times gone by monasteries were a good place for investigating the world inside. They were places where one was relatively free from the worries and cares in the world outside. You had a roof over your head and food on your plate. And your work was typically limited to meditative tasks such as chopping wood and carrying water. Today our practice time - whether that is at home in our living room or at a class in the local studio - is our monastery time. It is our time for going inside and, metaphorically speaking, our time for chopping wood and carrying water.

The yoga of the Yoga Sutras is also generally considered to be a scientific approach to yoga. Firstly, because the yoga of the Yoga Sutras uses the tool of reductionism to support us in building connection, to support us in dissolving separation. From just a summary reading of the Yoga Sutras we can see that a substantial part of the text is made up of lists. A telltale sign of reductionism at work. And secondly because the frameworks and tools presented in the text are based on the repeated experiments of the yogis of old; these are frameworks based on their common experience.

The Yoga Sutras is also a text that many of us struggle with for a while. We may find it dry and abstract, and we may struggle to find meaning and relevance to our yoga and our lives. So here is a short interpretation of the text. Very short, with a little sweetness, and in the language of our times: *There is this state of being, and we call it yoga, that is characterised by freedom, peace and joy. It is a limitless - and to be honest - pretty weird place. Take some time to hang out there; it is our home. You can either realise that now or you can do some work. When you choose to work, you might as well work in a specific way. In a way that will facilitate overcoming the obstacles you experience. Obstacles that all stem from the perspective that you are currently taking - that you don't really know who you are. Obstacles that manifest in all the patterns you appear to be caught up in. And, to get you on your way, here are a couple of methods you could use to overcome these obstacles.*

Although the Yoga Sutras is a text of great depth to which we can return time and time again it is also a very simple text. It is a simple text because it essentially covers just three themes: the Yoga Sutras describes the state of yoga; it discusses obstacles to yoga; and it offers a number of methods to move through the obstacles[14]. Only the text is not set out this way - it ducks and weaves coming at these three themes from different angles. It jumps from one theme to the other and it is a text that is direct and very indirect in its descriptions.

Mapping our obstacles. At the heart of the Yoga Sutras, stuck right between the state of yoga and methods to get there, is the idea of obstacles. To help us work in overcoming obstacles the yogis came up with the framework of the Kleshas. *The Kleshas are the five underlying obstacles that are postulated to give rise to all the individual patterns we find our selves caught up in.* This framework of the Kleshas is structured around a layering to these obstacles. The fundamental or root Klesha is Avidya, not knowing or ignorance of our true nature. Avidya gives rise to Asmita, egotism. Or in other words our stumbling around in the dark leads us to identify primarily with ego.

Layered on top of Avidya and Asmita are the three additional Kleshas. These are Raga, or attachment to pleasure, Dvesa, or aversion to pain, and Abhinivesah, or clinging to life out of fear of death. In the yogi's framework of the Kleshas these three give rise to the manifestation of all the games our ego-self gets caught up in. They give the colour to the patterns that define our experience: the thoughts we keep getting caught up in, the things we do by habit, the feelings we recycle and the energy states we get drawn to. The framework of the Kleshas is shown in the illustration below.

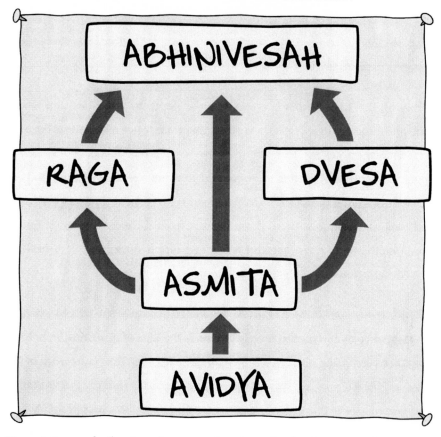

Now let's mesh the two frameworks given in the last two illustrations together in the context of our yoga on our mats. When we work and play in yoga from the perspective of the Yoga Sutras then we are in essence loosening our selves from obstacles and growing our ability to move towards, and remain in, a state of yoga. So we can place the state of yoga as the state box in the triggers, filters and states framework. We move towards this state in our practice times by turning our attention inside, and in doing so we reduce our exposure to and entanglement with internal triggers and triggers from our environment. We do this both by boxing off our practice time and by using specific methods and attitude - and we'll get a whole lot deeper into attitude in the next section. As we experience the triggers keep coming so we bring our attention back again and again.

What are left of course are the filters. We can see the whole Klesha framework as shedding light on the filters - on the sorting process that our automatic pilot carries out. Working down through the Kleshas framework from the top there are four observations we can make. Firstly we can frame the Klesha of Abhinivesah as the force that maintains attachment to the patterns we find our selves in. Abhinivesah is the force that clings to the known out of fear of the unknown. These patterns may manifest in different ways for each of us but they have in common that they are manifestations of the lower Kleshas. Secondly we can see the Kleshas of Raga and Dvesa as the two possible categories or boxes that a trigger can be allocated to. Simply put, we have a box for good and a box for bad. Good being attachment to pleasure and bad being aversion to pain. Although it may seem at times like the wiring got mixed up. And thirdly we can see Asmita - or egoism - as the architect of our boxes.

So when we frame it this way then we can see Raga and Dvesa as empty boxes, Asmita as that which defines each box by determining which box each trigger - or situation we find our selves in - is placed, and Abhinivesah makes sure we behave according to one of the patterns allocated to that box. *In the framework of the Kleshas it is egoism or Asmita that plays the role of the proverbial ghost in the machine, supported by Abhinivesah playing the role our internal forces of law and order.*

Which brings us on to our fourth observation and this is where the yogi's framework of the Kleshas begins to get really juicy. This is where yoga as a system for personal empowerment begins to really kick in. The fourth observation centres on the root Klesha of Avidya. As we saw earlier Avidya is ignorance of our true nature and etymologically speaking Avidya is the negation - that is the a at the beginning of the word - of Vidya. And Vidya means knowledge and specifically the knowledge from seeing things clearly. *Thus we can frame ignorance of our true nature as not seeing - our not seeing reality as it is.* A not seeing that locks us into the perspective of egoism and all that brings.

Now the option to identify with ego is a good thing: without ego we would not last very long. So contrary to popular belief yoga, and with it the other disciplines of the East, is not about getting rid of ego. Rather the practice of yoga is one of loosening the grip of ego on how we experience life. Yoga is a practice of creating the space to allow other perspectives of self to arise. This is the space we create through our work and play in yoga on our mat, and the space that allows for the opportunity for the four higher Kleshas in the yogi's framework to move up to in the light. It is the space that brings the play of Asmita, Raga, Dvesa and Abhinivesah into the seen. By bringing this play into the light we literally clean up our filters - our lenses of perception - and we rub up against and grow our experience of reality as it is. We experience reality unclouded by the distortions effected by egoism and its plays. Through this we diminish our pool of ignorance of our true nature. This is yoga as a system for personal empowerment.

This is probably a good point to remind our selves again that a framework is just a framework, and that this is therefore not the only way to frame the yogi's idea of the Kleshas. We could also frame the higher Kleshas as states we find our selves in. However framing the Kleshas as filters in this way is powerful because it links a framework, which although central to the Yoga Sutras can seem abstract and of little relevance, to the much simpler framework of triggers, filters and states. This simpler framework we can all directly relate to common situations we find our selves in and to our everyday behaviours. Framing the Kleshas in this way is also aligned with one of the central ideas in the Yoga Sutras that what stands between each of us and the state of yoga are the vacillating waves of perception - what is going on in our heads. *Stepping back from this discussion what is key in this whole section is the idea that we practice yoga to loosen our selves from the patterns we've become entangled in.* Practice that in essence functions to bring these patterns up into the light where we can see them.

When we practice yoga we work and play with the only thing we have: our own experience. For most of us this experience is most immediately coloured by what is closest to the surface. This is our entry point in our explorations and this is where we begin to bring the unseen into the seen. And the way loosening from pattern works for most of us, most of the time, is that we move through gross to subtle. We move from the patterns that are near the surface to those that run deep. As a general rule the deeper we go the more enticing our work and play becomes, and the greater the potential for change. Simply because the more subtle the pattern, the deeper that pattern runs in our being, the stronger the hold it has on us.

Allow surrender. In India they tell a story about how they train elephants to stay in one place. When the elephant is young they tether it to a stake with a thick rope. This rope is thick enough to hold the full force of the young elephant as it tries to break free. As the elephant gets older, and gets accustomed to the rope, they replace the thick rope with a thinner one. They can do this because the elephant no longer uses all its force to try to move away from the stake. The conditioning is beginning to get a hold on the elephant's behaviour. This process is repeated until the elephant is tethered with just a thin piece of string. This thin piece of string serves as a subtle reminder that keeps the full-grown elephant in place.

This is where the traditional story ends. However if you follow the news from India you know there is more: every once in a while a full-grown elephant loses it, breaks free, and runs amok through the local villages causing havoc. Taking both the original story and the unintended collateral damage we can conclude that the elephant's options appear to be limited to two: submitting to conditioning or running wild.

Yoga offers us an option the elephant does not have. Because when we work and play with the tools of yoga we bring our own thin pieces of string into the light. We bring the stuff that is messing with our perception of experience out of the shadows and observe them. And the yogic framework of the Kleshas gives us an entry point for our patterns, for our pieces of string: our likes and dislikes. So from awareness we get curious about our patterns of likes and dislikes and we observe them. *And through allowing our selves to observe them as they are - to see them and just let them be - we let go and disengage from them.*

Joining the Dots

Attitude and method. This is where the rubber hits the road, where our yoga gets up real close and personal. *Because when we practice yoga in a way that is radically simple on our mats we each investigate our own experience. We open our selves to the exploration of how patterns manifest in our own experience.* We are not exploring the experience of our teacher, not the experience of the authors of any books we may read, not exploring anybody else's experience but our own. This is the heart of the invitation of the yoga of going inside, the yoga of the Yoga Sutras.

When we practice the yoga of going inside we in essence place a little container around our experience. In our practice time we leave our beliefs, rules, our preconceptions of what is, outside that container. Perhaps most importantly we leave our self-striving outside the container. Then we turn up the heat - very literally in some forms of mat-based yoga - and we drop down the rabbit hole into the mystery of self. We drop into the fertile ground of our exploration.

So we don't take much with us when we go down. We don't need much stuff: in this sense yoga is a kit-light practice. *What we do take is our attitude to practice and method.* By method we mean the techniques associated with the particular style or form of yoga we are practicing. The different methods impact in different ways on our physical and energetic systems, and whilst there are good reasons from this perspective for choosing one method over another when it comes to radically simple yoga the specifics of the style or form of yoga we practice are irrelevant. So we are not going to delve into the details of technique here. We are going to keep it simple and radical. We will restrict our discussion of method to the root that supports all technique - our relationship with breath. And method at the level of breath and our attitude to practice are intimately intertwined. We cannot pull them apart and label our relationship with breath and our attitude as separate things.

So to explore and grow our insight into attitude and method here we are going to approach them from different angles. We will start by looking at our belly, head and heart on our mats. Then we will look at balance and flow. And we will conclude by exploring the mysterious practice of non-violence.

Our belly, head and heart on our mats: The Yoga Sutras of Patanjali have a lot to say about our attitude to practice. Attitude is included - albeit sometimes obscurely - in all the methods suggested in the text. Here we are going to look at attitude as encapsulated in the method of Kriya Yoga. This is the method we looked at briefly in Chapter Two when we introduced our philosopher's anatomy of belly, head and heart. And Kriya Yoga comprises the three practices of Tapah, Svadhyaya and Isvara-Pranidhana. Or in plain English the practice of dedication to, and purification through, practice; the practice of self-study; and the practice of surrender to what is. These practices are rooted in our bellies, heads and hearts. Three practices that in essence are one practice. One practice that we pull apart to frame, structure, communicate and give us something to work with. Three parts that we reintegrate in each moment when we roll out our mats and practice.

The practice of Tapah is our commitment to practice. Tapah is a commitment to the means, the process, of practice and a commitment that has nothing to do with the results of practice. It is a commitment that is rooted in our belly - it is our will realised in action. *So when we practice mat-based physical yoga we commit to that practice without concern for results. This is our attitude of belly.* So in mat-based yoga the question is not: *'how can I progress in this posture?'* Rather the focus for our curiosity is: *'what is going on for me in this posture right now?'* We direct our effort of awareness to our experience in the present moment. And the sweet thing is that when we sustain this effort of attention then we will bear fruit, we will undergo transformation.

Svadhyaya, the second practice of Kriya Yoga, is study - and first and foremost the study of self. Self is what we work with in yoga. In many forms of yoga Svadhyaya often extends to the study of the core texts of yoga. The core texts that explore the key ideas in yoga, and provide a context for the system of yoga that may be useful. The central and most important step in study is observation. To grow our ability to observe means we grow our ability to use our awareness to direct our attention. We direct the attention that lives throughout our being. This is an ability that is rooted in our head.

When it comes to mat-based yoga applying observation means integrating the practice of Svadhyaya with that of Tapah. Thus when we engage in the physical practices of yoga we develop the ability to adopt both the perspective of the one practicing and the one observing the one practicing. This is how we develop discrimination. This discrimination plays out at many levels: in working out how to practice Asana that is both safe and functional for us, in finding and exploring our edge, in distinguishing between experience and our reaction or response to experience, and so on. This is discrimination that flows from our seeing what is, from bringing our filters up into the light and in doing so loosening our selves from their grip. *This is discrimination that is rooted in self-observation in the present moment. This is our attitude of head.*

The third practice of Kriya yoga is Isvara-Pranidhana, the practice of surrender. Or more accurately surrender to the Lord. Which sounds good when you are into Lords - or Ladies - and surrendering to them is your thing. When we are not it is also good. *Because the key thing here is surrender.* And surrendering means easing off that tight little grip we hold on our reality, easing off the control button. It is about opening up to experience and accepting what comes. When it comes to our mat-based yoga the practice of surrender goes hand in hand with the practices of Tapah and of Svadhyaya. *It is a practice of surrender that flows with our dedication to practice and of seeing things as they are. It is a practice of opening up to this present moment in this present moment. This is our attitude of heart.*

Our attitude of belly, head and heart can only be manifested in each present moment. *We can only manifest dedication now and we can only see and open up to what is now.* It is being here in this present moment that forges the three practices of Kriya Yoga into one practice, that moves us from practicing yoga to engaging with the state of yoga. So when we roll out our mats, and put that little container around our experience, we practice, we observe and we surrender. We ease off on the interfering and we grow our ability to observe and accept what comes up as we go down into our selves. We practice - Tapah. We take a good look at our selves, a really good look at our selves, again and again. This is our Svadhyaya. And we ride and surrender to the balance and flow of that which arises with love and acceptance - Isvara-Pranidhana. Which brings us on to balance and flow.

Balance and flow is the essence of yoga on our mats. Balance and flow is the essence of our practice of yoga Asana, or yoga postures, which for many in the West today is yoga. And there are many forms of Asana practice. All of which work in a manifold of ways on our physical and energetic bodies. At one end of the spectrum we have the overtly active - or Yang - forms of practice such as the Vinyasa forms, Ashtanga yoga, and other flow forms. At the other end there are the more passive - or Yin - forms of practice, such as Yin yoga and restorative yoga. And there is everything in between.

Although these forms may look, may seem and may feel very different they are all practices of Tapah. They are practices of purification or loosening our selves from the grip of the Kleshas, practices we engage in from our attitude of belly, head and heart. And to uncover the essence of Asana practice we turn again to the Yoga Sutras. The Yoga Sutras are made up of 196 verses and exactly two of these are dedicated to the physical practice of Asana. It took just two verses for the yogis of old to convey the posture part of yoga on our mats. So those two verses must be pretty important.

The first of these, Sutra II-46, defines Asana and reads: "*Yoga pose is a steady and comfortable position.*"[15] Now whilst this Sutra is very short it contains two messages. *Firstly Asana is characterised in terms of both an active, or doing component and a passive, or non-doing component.* This doing component, here translated as steadiness, can also be framed as alertness, firmness, or something similar. The non-doing component, here translated as comfortable, can also be framed as relaxed, easy, or something similar. *The second message contained in this Sutra is the idea or implication of some sort of balance between doing and non-doing.*

Mind being as it is has the tendency to grasp for some sort of understanding of balance. Our minds fall for the temptation to conceive of balance as a static quality. Balance however is slippery - the moment we try to grasp balance it shifts. This is one of the common experiences we all have when we practice Asana. And the next sutra, Sutra II-47, sheds a little light on this.

Sutra II-47 describes how to master Asana - how to grow our ability and experience in Asana. Or in other words this Sutra outlines how to explore balance between doing and non-doing: "*Yoga pose is mastered by relaxation of effort, lessening of the tendency for restless breathing, and promoting an identification of oneself as living within the infinite breath of life.*" Again there are a couple of messages contained within this Sutra. The first message is one that is very opportune for many of us in the West, for those of us who have been conditioned by the efficiency machine. *And that message is let go; ease off our automatic doing.* So the challenge for each of us in this message is to become aware of how doing is most colouring our own experience: in our doing, our thinking and our feeling, and in how we are engaging energetically with reality as it unfolds. This is the heart of our Svadhyaya on the mat.

Letting go of something is one part of letting go. The other part is letting go into something. This is the second message contained in Sutra II-47: *we let go into the infinite; we let go into the flow of breath.* And as we let go into, and move our experience into, the flow of breath, this is where we explore balance. Or in other words, the balance between doing and non-doing rides the flow of breath. It is breath that is the foundation of, and the guide for, our practice. Surrendering to, and finding balance on, the flow of the breath is the heart of our Isvara-Pranidhana on the mat.

Our practice on our mats is practice for life and life is relationship: our life plays out in, and is defined by, relationship with, everything around us. It is in relationship that our belly finds purpose, our hearts express love, and our head grows wisdom. In the old worldview of separation relationship is characterised by comparison - better than, bigger than, in debt to, that sort of thing. This is simply because when there is more than one then comparison creeps in. In the worldview of connection, relationship is characterised by balance and flow: balance and flow, here and now.

We have covered a lot of ground in this chapter. We have looked at our practice of yoga on our mats as an invitation to heal our selves. We framed yoga as practice for loosening our selves from entanglement in patterns that reinforce an illusion of separation. We then introduced a simple model of triggers, filters and states to frame how we become entangled in pattern. And we have seen how we can frame the yogi's idea of the Kleshas - the basic obstacles that manifest in pattern - so as to shed light on how our filters function. We have seen that when we practice yoga on our mats we are in essence engaging in an exploration of our own experience. Experience that is coloured in whatever way patterns manifest with us. And we have discussed how, whatever the form or style of yoga we are practicing, we bring our attitude of belly, head and heart to this exploration - attitude that is rooted in the now. And lastly we explored the centrality of breath in method in our yoga practice: of our yoga practice being one of riding and surrendering into the balance and flow of breath as it manifests in each moment. Now it is time to pull this all together, and we will do this by exploring non-violence.

Non-violence permeates and empowers our yoga practice. Non-violence permeates our practice because our attitude to practice is non-violent and our method of grounding in breath is non-violent. When non-violence permeates our practice it then empowers our practice in two very specific ways. Casting our minds back to our framework of triggers, filters and state we can recall that we are generally aware of the triggers and the state: these are in the seen. In contrast the filters are generally out of our line of sight: they are in the unseen. So the first way in which our non-violent attitude and method empower our practice is that they allow for the space to arise where there is the opportunity for that which is unseen to become seen. The creation of this space allows that which is in the shadow to move into the light.

Secondly it is our non-violent attitude and method that takes us towards, and then time and time again back towards, a state of yoga and away from our habitual reactive states. So it is the infusing of our attitude and method with non-violence that empowers our yoga practice. *It is non-violence that provides the fertile ground for the two effects described above to take seed, to grow and to blossom.* Or in other words we cannot force the space for the Kleshas to unfold into the seen and we cannot force our selves into a state of yoga. These two effects of attitude and method are shown in the illustration below.

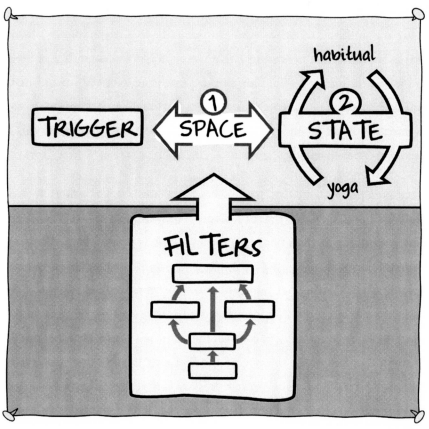

Non-violence, known in yoga as Ahimsa, is explicitly covered in the Yoga Sutras as the first of the Yamas. The Yamas are the moral code or guidelines within the method of Ashtanga. Probably for this reason Ahimsa is often broken down to a set of rules or guidelines: guidelines such as don't hurt others or your self, don't eat meat, or don't speak harmful words. *Ahimsa is however a practice, and Ahimsa is a much more mysterious practice than one that can be codified in rules.* Ahimsa permeates all the yoga philosophy texts, as well as the Taoist thinking from China.

It is Ahimsa that empowers our practices of Tapah, Svadhyaya and Isvara-Pranidhana. When we leave our self-striving outside the container of our practice then we create the conditions for gentleness towards our selves to unfold. When we practice with gentleness then we create the conditions for ever deeper seeing without interfering. *Because one thing we can take from our simple framework of triggers, filters and states is that when we are stuck in habitual mode we are always doing something to our selves.* A doing that is driven by our egoism. So our Svadhyaya becomes an ever deeper seeing without engaging our automatic pilot and succumbing to pattern. And our ever deeper seeing without interfering creates the conditions for surrender to what we are seeing. Because one thing we can take from the yogi's framework of the Kleshas is that there is a ground of being beyond egoism. *That mysterious ground of being where not doing something to our selves becomes an option.* So our Isvara-Pranidhana becomes a surrendering into the unfolding mystery of self-knowledge. Ultimately it is Ahimsa that fuses the three practices of belly, head and heart into one practice of being. It is through Ahimsa that we let go and move beyond our frameworks of belly, head and heart and of our practices of Tapah, Svadhyaya and Isvara-Pranidhana.

And it is Ahimsa that guides and empowers our exploration of the balance and flow of breath. Simply because Ahimsa starts with every breath we breathe - or with every breath that we receive. As we deepen our relationship with breath we create the conditions to allow our selves to drop ever deeper down into the rabbit hole of self. *Ahimsa takes the light of our awareness ever down into what was the unseen - into the shadow places in our being.* So from this perspective yoga is an original form of shadow work. Which brings us to yet another thing that some modern Western thinkers and the yogis of old agree on: we cannot dissolve shadow with mind. It is through the practices of non-violent attitude and method - practices that move us beyond mind - that we clean our filters. We clean the lenses of perception that our ego mind installs and maintains. These practices take us deeper into the recesses of our being and towards a greater sense of self, of truth.

The power and potential of attitude and method of the yoga of the Yoga Sutras - the yoga of going inside - is that it joins the dots. It grows connection. As we practice we work and play with the only thing we have: our own experience and the patterns that limit this. We bring these patterns into the light where we can see them. We bring them from the unseen to the seen. And as we get real up close and intimate to our own patterns one of the things we experience is that they are related to each other. *We experience that the things we had separated out and labelled with little words, such as mind, emotion, body, breath, are actually deeply interconnected.* Through this radically simple approach to the practice of yoga on our mats we experience that the belief in separation just does not hold up in our own being.

As we dissolve the illusion of separation in our own being we begin to realise for our selves the message of the Yoga Sutras: heal your self, rediscover your wholeness. We realign our selves through a realignment of our belly, hearts and heads. We realign our selves at an energetic level. At a deep and subtle level we start joining the dots that science cannot join. *This is yoga as a spiritual practice, as reconnection with spirit.* This is yoga that opens our hearts in a very real way: it grows our ability to enjoy our experience even when we don't like what is going on. When we touch base with that mysterious ground of being inside, that space that gifts us peace and joy, the more able we are to ride out the rough times in our lives. It is not that those times necessarily become any easier but we do face those times with connection to our true source of strength.

It is through our work and play of loosening from pattern that we start to realise for our selves and in our own being a shift from the old story of separation towards the new story of connection. This ultimately is the power and beauty of the gift of the yoga of the Yoga Sutras. Engaging with this gift through attitude and breath infused with non-violence is yoga made real in action.

Inner Prop: Allow Surrender

The Prop: Allowing surrender means seeing and accepting what is. Really accepting means accepting with our Whole Being. And through accepting we melt into what is. Surrender is an ever deeper letting go of that tight grip we all hold on reality. A grip we hold because we have been conditioned to believe we have to. It is a grip that we hold in different ways, and we hold way down deep into our being. This belief that holds us stems from fear - the fear that letting go of that grip is the end. Yoga invites us to entertain otherwise - that letting go of that grip really is the beginning.

If there is one prop that can really support us in the West then it is the prop of surrender. Because we have been deeply conditioned into doing - we have become chronic doers, we do all the time. We do with our bellies, we do with our heads and we do with our hearts. And we do energetically so that our being has become doing. This is one very real and central part of the damage inflicted upon us as individuals by living within the old story of separation. Because doing is all there is left in the material world when we take away spirit, spirit that rides the breath of life.

The Prop of Surrender on our Mats: **Our mat-based yoga practice is one of surrender rather than striving.** Through practice we grow our ability to follow the subtle way of non-violence. And whatever style or form of yoga we practice on our mats it is breath that guides us ever deeper into surrender. That is, our physical movement is secondary to the breath movement and *'the body movement is encapsulated within the breath movement.'*[16] And when we practice yoga on our mats it is the breath movement that guides us in finding our edge, our balance between doing and non-doing, and that guides our practice in a way that is safe and functional.

Observing and surrendering to breath is an ongoing practice. It is a practice that shifts what we tend to think of as a physical practice - yoga Asana on our mats - towards an energetic practice. *And it is the core practice in which we explore what surrender means for each of us.* Surrender in the form of observing what is - the practice of just seeing or just listening, not only with our eyes and ears but also with our whole being. This is a practice of observing without intervening: observing our thoughts and our doing, observing the ups and the downs of our emotional journey, and observing how we feel energetically.

This is also surrender in the form of exploring how to distinguish between functional and non-functional doing. Where functional is defined by each of us in the context of how we fill whatever form our practice takes. Through growing our ability to make this distinction we can strengthen our functional doing through intent realised with will in action. And we can ease off the non-functional doing in our being. As we move deeper our surrender takes the form of connecting, merging and balancing our observing, feeling and doing. We grow the connection in our belly, head and heart in spirit as we ride the flow of breath.

Many of us in the West come to yoga to relax. We come for that feeling of relaxation at the end of practice. And in this respect our yoga delivers. So yoga fills a need because if there is one pattern that really is endemic in the West it is that of stress. *When we practice radically simple yoga we grow our ability to start our practice from a position of openness, a position of relaxation.* So when we roll out our mats we take the time to breathe. We breathe deep into our belly, into our being, to centre and to ground. In short, we come into our being. And from that position of openness we start to practice. We explore surrender from a position of relaxation.

The Prop of Surrender in our Worlds: Surrender in our world is a challenge. It is a challenge because it is in our world that we go out and do. And it is a challenge because we are conditioned - both internally and externally - to equate doing with achievement. We tend to do until we collapse, and collapsing is very different to surrender. Surrender in our world flows from curiosity with our growth in awareness. Because our curiosity grows our ability to see things how they are. Once we see things as they are we can begin to discriminate, to formulate intention, and realise our intention through will in action. And this realisation can manifest as a going out and doing something or it can manifest as surrender.

When we apply surrender to our everyday lives off our mats we explore where to ease off. And a good starting point is that well-known rule of thumb: *"Change what you cannot accept. Accept what you cannot change."*[17] This is a starting point because there is a big grey area between these two. *In that grey area - and in analogy to our practice on our mats - lies our edge.* When we stay well within our edge, within our comfort zone, our surrendering is conforming to pattern, to habit. When we move with intentional action and rub up against our edge then our surrendering becomes accepting of what is. This is the surrendering that fosters change. This is the surrendering that is the cornerstone of non-violent personal evolution.

One of the big patterns we find our selves entangled in is looking back into our past. A pattern that - whatever its uses and attractions - often serves to reinforce the narrative that our egoism creates and recreates to define us as a person. This narrative often places us as a victim of circumstance - the subject of stuff done to us by others and the world. The yogis of old postulate that rather than analyse and story-tell about our past we surrender to what is now, and a powerful practice for this is forgiveness. So we practice forgiveness towards our selves, forgiveness towards others, and forgiveness towards the world. As our practice of yoga deepens so does our practice of forgiveness. Our practice of forgiveness shifts towards a practice of radical forgiveness: a sinking deeper into the realisation that there is no thing and no one to forgive.

4. Stuff and Distractions

Our yoga turns the spotlight of our attention to how we habitually colour our own experience. To our patterns of belly, head and heart, and to what distracts us. Focus brings us back time and time again to our work and play at hand, right here and now.

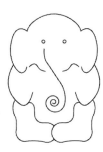

Common Patterns

Exploring the flip side. One of the things we all experience when we practice yoga is that all sorts of stuff comes up. From one perspective this is most definitely our stuff: stuff that is deeply personal and stuff we all work and play with. This work and play brings to each of us our own opportunities and our own challenges. *From another perspective, and whilst recognising that we are each going to go through this in our own sweet way, there is most definitely a pattern to our patterns.* That, in the language of the simple framework of triggers, filters and states used in the previous chapter, there is a pattern to the common states of being that we all find our selves in. This should not surprise us as we are all subject to the same evolutionary constraints and have all been deeply conditioned by the same basic tenets of the old story. In this section we are going to look at the patterns to the stuff that comes up - common patterns.

We are going to start with what we will call exploring the flip side. We will explore patterns of belly, head and heart that can be framed as the opposite of the yoga practices of Tapah, Svadhyaya and Isvara-Pranidhana that we covered in the previous chapter. Then we will build on this by looking at the pattern of stress. A pattern that is endemic in our modern world. And then we will move on to the patterns of fear and laziness. In the next section we will move on to explore a different sort of common pattern: red herrings, or things that distract us from our yoga.

Attitude is key in yoga and yoga provides us with attitude skills of belly, head and heart to disentangle from pattern and to make our yoga real. These are the attitude skills of Tapah, Svadhyaya and Isvara-Pranidhana that we explored in detail in the previous chapter. Now what many of us discover when we practice yoga is that our habitual attitude of belly, head and heart can be framed as the flip side of the attitude skills required in yoga. We will call these flip sides the Doing Machine, the Story Teller and the Drama Trip. These flip side patterns are shown in the illustration below.

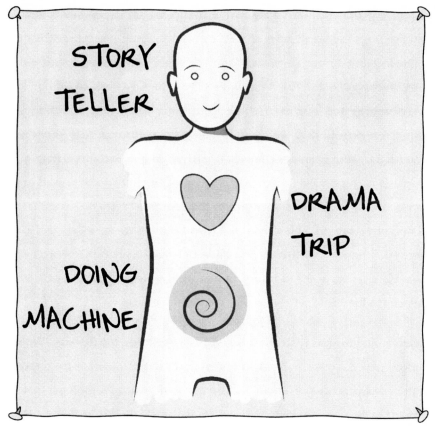

The Doing Machine is a pattern of chronic doing that has nestled itself deep into our being. This is a pattern that is relentless in its focus on completion of one thing and moving on to the next. *The Doing Machine is characterised by an attitude that is result focused and operates - often literally - by ticking things off lists.* When we are entangled in the Doing Machine we are never fully present. Our attention is never fully in the now unfolding. Entanglement in the Doing Machine messes with our Tapah - our engagement with action in each moment for the sake of that action.

Entanglement with the Doing Machine is part and parcel of the old story of separation. In this story we have been reduced to the role of cogs in the efficiency machine of the material. We are given something to do and instructions on how to do it. We have become cogs that are both incentivised and goaded to spin a little faster, and then a little faster again. Disentanglement from the Doing Machine starts with getting curious about chronic doing in our being. And although we have framed this chronic doing as rooted in our belly it may manifest in any and all parts of our system. As we get curious about this chronic doing our yoga practice brings this into the light so that our curiosity deepens our seeing. Loosening from the Doing Machine follows from this ever deeper seeing combined with bringing our selves back again and again to the attitude of Tapah.

The Story Teller is the lover of narrative. It is that part of mind that latches on to some thought - often some memory or future fantasy - which then leads to another thought. The Story Teller takes these thoughts, attaches some sort of significance to them, and then strings them together into some sort of narrative. This narrative then comes to somehow define our persona, it defines us as a person and drives our behaviours. The Story Teller creates narratives that are largely driven by judgement and labels, by good and bad, by desires and disappointments. In other words, it is the Kleshas of Raga and Dvesa that form the contextual box for our patterns of behaviour.

These narratives are captivating. *We get riveted to, and identify with, the narrative the Story Teller is constructing.* Whilst the narrative captivates our attention it becomes our reality: it is more real to us than what is going on in the here and now, in our bodies and in the space around us. *When we are entangled in the pattern of the Story Teller our attitude is largely in the past or future and characterised by judgement.* When the Story Teller looms large in our experience this is going to mess big time with our ability to observe and to accept what is. It is going to mess with our attitude practice of Svadhyaya.

The yogis of old gave a lot of attention to thought and they postulated that everything comes back to consciousness. *For the yogi consciousness is primary and the material world is birthed from this deeper reality.* The yogis postulated that our link to this primary reality is mind. And they framed our mind as having three parts. We can see the Story Teller as akin to that part of mind the yogis called Ahamkara, or the I-maker. The thoughts that the Story Teller locks into become actions in the material world. Actions repeated become habit, habit hardened becomes character, and character locked in becomes destiny. So although we have framed the Story Teller as a pattern rooted in our heads this is a pattern that - just like the Doing Machine - has wormed itself into all parts of our being.

A common manifestation of the flip side of Svadhyaya is the Story Teller getting stuck. The Story Teller going around and around in circles of its own making. We experience this commonly when our rational mind runs up against something beyond its understanding. Now our rational problem-solving mind is one of our great developments in evolution. *However when it runs up against a wall and leads us in a merry dance round and round in circles it becomes a hindrance and not an asset.* In essence our mind becomes an Idiot Box. When we are in the grip of the Idiot Box we will experience this on and off our mats with rational mind jumping in to claim a piece of the action. We can see the Idiot Box as the flip side of the second part of the yogi's three-part framework of mind - Buddhi or the discriminative function of mind. When we are entangled in the Idiot Box we get stuck. We get caught up in analysing rather than observing and discriminating.

When we are entangled in the Drama Trip we are in the grip of the rollercoaster of our emotions. In many cases this rollercoaster is powered by what are often labelled negative emotions and the tendency to play victim. These emotional patterns are - from the perspective of modern science - associated with the release of a specific set of neuropeptides from the hypothalamus in our brain. The neuropeptides then attach to cells all over our bodies inducing a particular reaction in those cells. We can relate the Drama Trip to the third part of the yogi's three-part framework of mind - Manas or the desiring part of mind. *The Drama Trip is Manas magnified and manifesting as the omnipresent author of the heaven and hell of our own making. When we are entangled in the Drama Trip the pattern is often one of resistance.* When we are caught up superimposing heaven and hell on our experience, and caught up in resistance, this is going to mess with our practice of Isvara-Pranidhana, our practice of surrendering to what is.

Now we may not immediately see our stuff that comes up in terms of the Doing Machine, the Story Teller or the Drama Trip. After all this is just a framework and the lens to look at a framework is one of usefulness not truth. So it may be that this framework of patterns to the flip side of yoga simply does not resonate for us - it does not fulfil its purpose of usefulness. Or it may be because we are all stressed out. And when we are all stressed out then our ability to see is - very literally - restricted: stress limits us in seeing our stuff as it is. So let us turn to look at stress.

All stressed out. We all experience stress to some extent. Stress is part of life - it is our natural reaction to certain situations. *However our modern world and lifestyles accentuate this reaction to the degree that if there is one pattern endemic today it is that of chronic stress.* And one of the tricky things about stress is that it is good at hiding. This is because our nervous system works on so-called change messages - it registers and reacts to changes in our system. So that if we chronically sustain a higher level of stress our nervous system takes this as the new normal. It is only when our stress becomes even higher that it notices change.

Our framework of belly, head and heart provides a useful starting point for exploring how the pattern of stress manifests. And by exploring - and through exploring just seeing - beginning to loosen from that pattern. Simply because most of us verbalise our experience of stress in one or more of these three areas: in our physical body - our belly as a feeling of tightness, or tension in our hips, neck or shoulders; in our heads - the incessant chatter of repetitive thoughts; in our hearts or emotionally - we become prickly and easily upset. In addition we may experience it more holistically, as a feeling of agitation or unrest in our being as a whole.

However we experience it we all have one thing in common. *Our stress is a pulling tight or closing in somewhere in our system.* That is very literally - because stress comes from the Latin word stressare which means to pull tight - what stress does to us. This pulling tight restricts our vision, our ability to see things as they are. *In this way stress impacts our experience of the world because this experience depends on the state of our nervous system.* So by pulling tight stress restricts our options for response - it reduces our self response-ability. And to come back to where we started stress is also a root pattern: besides the pattern of pulling tight, locking into stress locks us into all sorts of behaviour patterns - patterns of doing, thinking patterns and emotional patterns. As a consequence of stress we may not be able to see the other patterns we are entangled in. So when we practice to loosen from pattern then a very good strategy is to start with the pattern of stress.

As we saw in Chapter One many of us discover yoga when we want to de-stress. This is our motivation for practice: we take our first yoga class because we have heard that it is great for relaxation. And it is - it works! It works both in and of itself, for example when we experience that feeling of total-being relaxation after a fast-flowing Vinyasa class. We learn that a little directional effort makes the surrender into relaxation just that little bit sweeter. And it works through paying specific attention to where we feel tension in our physical bodies, for example in a Yin class. We keep coming back for more. *Here lies a danger because another common pattern - and one that by its very nature is specific to yoga - is the pattern of yoga as a pill.* This is the pattern of using our yoga practice as our weekly or daily pill to relax from the stresses of the rest of our life. And as long as we are using yoga as a pill for stress then we run the very real risk of getting stuck. We become stuck in a cycle of loosening and then re-tightening our relationship with stress. We become stuck in never creating the sustainable space to move beyond the pattern of stress. When we are stuck here then yoga, as a system for personal empowerment, is just not going to kick in. Which brings us on to two more common patterns.

Tracking down fear and laziness. The fear and laziness we are going to explore here have no moral judgements attached - at least certainly not at our individual level. Fear and laziness are tendencies that are played upon, manipulated, and amplified by the old story to keep us in our box, to keep us in our place. *So odds on, once we start practicing yoga in a way that is radically simple - in a way that is specifically designed to empower us to move out of that box - we are going to run up against fear and we are going to run up against laziness.*

We run up against fear because in the world of separation we have been conditioned to behave as if the only thing that holds us together are our patterns of likes and dislikes. This is the yogi's framework of the Kleshas in action and amplified by the subtle and not-so-subtle programming of our modern world. Our ego-self clings on to pleasure and runs from pain out of fear of its death. Our practice of yoga brings this behaviour into the light; we begin to see it for what it is. We see how we are boxed in and fear kicks in. This fear is very different to the fear that may kick in when we get a signal that we might be about to injure our self by pushing into a posture when our body is saying no. The fear we experience as we rub up against what boxes us in is a sign that our yoga is starting to get real.

This is the fear that we sit with. And as we sit with it, the fear dissipates and allows us to drop deeper: as the fear dissipates it takes with it a layer of entanglement in pattern. So when we embark on healing we move beyond the limits imposed by the illusion of separation. We move into the unknown. And feeling a little fear when we move into the unknown is a good thing. It keeps us alert. It is through feeling the fear and moving into the unknown that we build courage.

Where we run up against this fear we may also run up against laziness. This laziness is - just like fear - part and parcel of the world of separation. Part and parcel because the world of separation places value on efficiency: with the belief in separation comes the efficiency machine. And the efficiency machine works like this: through patterns we come to believe in repetition. Or rather we get caught up in the illusion of repetition. This illusion stops us from observing what is; it is an illusion that locks us into a choice of perspective. Whatever the nature of the pattern, and whether it is a pattern that works for us or not, we choose perspective on automatic pilot. This automatic doing is the core of the efficiency machine. And automatic doing - whatever its place - comes with a price tag: the opportunity missed to open to the unique and wondrous magic of each present moment. The price we pay is authentic personal experience.

So the yoga of the Yoga Sutras requires work. It requires work to sit with our fear and work to loosen our selves from laziness. We work to counter all that functions to bring us back in our box, back into our comfort zone. We work to focus on, and listen to, the intelligence of our being speaking to us through fear. Because, without that work we turn back to what we know, we turn back to our confinement within pattern. We may even drop yoga for a while, our ego-self telling us that our yoga is not good for us and we should try something else.

So the work that yoga requires is not just the rolling out of our mats and our physical practice of Tapah. Our work involves growing our skills of Svadhyaya, self-study or self-observation, and Isvara-Pranidhana, acceptance or surrender. *And these skills are something we can all develop. To develop these we focus - during our practice time - on certain sets of behaviours.* We work and play to develop focused intention and observation. We work and play to grow our ability to let go, to ease off the tight little grip we hold on reality, to be with what is. Through this ongoing work and play we overcome our tendencies of laziness and fear, tendencies that dull our curiosity and that weaken the force of our awareness. We engage with the invitation of yoga to realise that this moment is happening for the very first time. And in this moment we all have space for choice - the choice of resorting to pattern or seeing and being with what is.

Our entry point for this work is what is most manifest in our own experience. The yoga of the Yoga Sutras provides a framework for the attitude skills of belly, head and heart for this work. This same framework also supports us in framing some of the common patterns - what we have called our flip side patterns. *Ultimately however our own experience is what we as individuals work with: simply because it is the only thing we have.* Our experience is real in a way that a framework never can be, and our practice of yoga mandates that we get real close and intimate with the realness of this experience. And this requires focus.

Maintain focus. When it comes to the world of connection the focus we are developing is that of a whole being focus. We are developing focus of mind, focus of heart, and focus of action. *Focus of our whole being on the work and play at hand: on growing our ability to see things as they are; on growing our ability to accept with ever deeper non-violence; and growing our ability to act from a place of wisdom and compassion.* We are developing focus in our practice on our mats and out in our world.

Our first and most important challenge when we engage in yoga practice is to let go of our motivation when we roll out our mat, when we step into our space for practice. At the very least taking our motivation for practice onto our mat is going to mess with our ability to observe, our ability to drop into the deeper space of self. This is the heart of the practice of Tapah on our mats and of Karma Yoga in our worlds. Of carrying out our work without expectation of, and attachment to, result. This is the knife-edge between something being useful and a distraction. So let's move on and look at some of the big distractions we may run up against.

Red Herrings and Other Attractive Fish

A red herring is a distraction. It is something that distracts or misleads us from our work at hand. *A red herring essentially captivates our attention and redirects the focus of our efforts.* There is only one little problem: no one has ever seen a red herring. As far as we know they may or may not exist. The term red herring is also applied for the literary technique of deliberately placing a decoy in a text to draw the readers towards a false conclusion. Or to something that is found in a text by the reader, a teacher or a tradition, that functions to distract us: this again is something that may or may not be there. So beware of thinking of the Yoga Sutras - or any book - as a sacred text. Sacred has the tendency to do something strange with mind. Or mind does something strange with sacred. Sacred often ends up on a pedestal.

There is nothing wrong with red herrings. How could there be something wrong with something that may or may not exist; or something right with them for that matter. Right and wrong are not the issue here. It is a question of when, and to what extent, something is useful. And however red herrings manifest they can provide a useful function. After all they may have been our doorway to yoga. They may be a part of our motivation for continuing to practice. As we saw back in Chapter One, any motivation for practice is good. It is good as long as it comes from inside, as long as we own it.

There is another very useful function that red herrings fulfil. They are a beautiful manifestation of connection within. They are an illustration of the illusion of separation because the grip of red herrings tends to run deep. Whatever form our red herrings take they have the tendency to bubble up and manifest throughout our system, throughout our experience - in our doing, in our feeling and in our thinking. In this way red herrings embody the truth that the deeper we delve into our experience the more we realise that our simple framework of belly, heart and head really is just a framework. That our doing, feeling and thinking are not just connected they are one: that any framework is just a framework.

Before we explore specific manifestations of red herrings in yoga let's look at what yoga has to say about the root of all red herrings. For that we turn again to the framework of the Kleshas that we explored in Chapter Three, and in particular to the root Klesha of Avidya. Avidya is not knowing or ignorance of our true nature and it is this ignorance that provides the fertile ground for all other obstacles. This includes all red herrings. Our mind is not keen on not knowing and the way mind functions, or is conditioned, to deal with this not knowing is to make assumptions. The mind seeks to turn not knowing into knowing. *We shift from the essence and uncertainty that are intimate to the mystery of self and life, to the illusion of safety in certainty.* As we do this we surround the dynamic heart of self, of life, of yoga, with a static shell. This is a shell that appears to be solid but is built on quicksand.

When we work with the practices of yoga as a system for empowerment then in one sense we engage in an exploration about who we are in the context of the mystery of reality. We work to uncover and loosen our selves from the play of mind in constructing static shells. So however we experience our red herrings the root of all red herrings is in our minds. When it comes to red herrings it is mind, and mind's tendency to grasp at knowing where we have locked down our choice of perspective. A locking down that limits our exploration of our true nature. Therefore to disentangle our selves from the grip of a red herring we bring the assumptions of mind from the unseen into the seen and check them out.

Right here, right now! Many of us come to yoga with the idea of getting there. We come with the idea of walking a path to get there or, at the very least, walking a path to get somewhere. *At some point yoga invites us to drop this and embrace the here and now.* This is shown below.

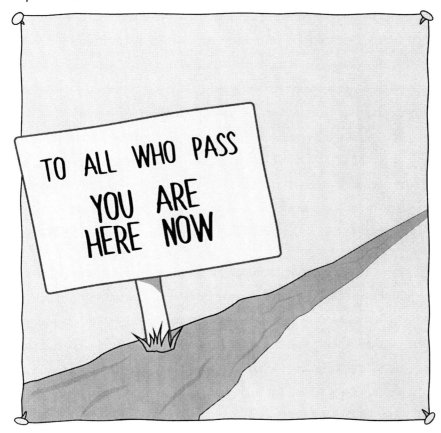

Getting there is one beautiful big red herring in yoga and getting there manifests as end-gaming. *This end-gaming stems from a focus on the idea of some kind of future situation that we project as being in some way complete, static and desirable.* It could be as down to earth as '*I want to feel relaxed after class*', as practical as '*I want to perfect this pose*' or as ambitious as '*I practice yoga to become enlightened*'. The common theme is a future situation that is different from where we find our selves now and that everything is going to be just fine when we get there. Entanglement in this red herring brings with it the flip side attitude of focus on results and goals often compounded with a pattern of competing with our selves.

In yoga today this red herring commonly manifests as physical getting there: as a focus on developing a healthier body or a body beautiful. It manifests as focus on a textbook proficiency in Asana practice or as a focus on mastering technique. Or it may manifest simply as desire for feeling relaxed after class. Again these are all good motivations to practice when we own them. It is when we take these onto the mat that they become red herrings: because our motivation filters up into our experience, it impacts our experience and distracts us from practice. When our motivation drives our practice as we practice it gets in the way of awareness, of curiosity, and of surrender. It distracts us from the exploration of our experience here and now. It distracts us from the heart of practice that is this present moment, a present moment that is just as it is, that is complete and inherently desirable.

The other common manifestation of the getting there red herring in yoga is a spiritual one. This is the red herring born of the sacred text put up on a pedestal. In yoga - as with many other spiritual traditions - this red herring is dressed up in the fine robes of the idea of enlightenment. This is an idea that our mind distils from what it has read and heard, projects onto our yoga and idealizes. This idea is characterised by a purity of seeing, being and doing that is complete and therefore static. When we practice yoga in a way that is radical and simple then we do not care so much about ideas as about experience. And in this respect our common experience is clear: whatever enlightenment is, and wherever we are right now, our work and our play goes on.

A second big beautiful red herring in yoga is walking a path, and when there is nowhere to get to what is the point of a path? *Paths are relics that pave the way between places in the land of separation.* Specifically when we walk a path in yoga sooner or later we experience one or both of the two following conundrums. Which are, of course, at their root one conundrum. Firstly, the deeper our yoga becomes the stronger the realisation that we step into mystery, into the unknown. There is no path there. This is when the path becomes the pathless path. And secondly, as we have all experienced on our mats and in our life, we keep going around in circles. We keep coming back to exactly where we are right now. We keep coming back to the here and now. Sure the backdrop or lighting may be a little different, however the essence is unchanged.

A common manifestation of walking a path in our mat-based yoga is taking refuge in the sanctuary of form, of a specific technique. Not that there is anything wrong with technique: in contrast, there are a lot of techniques that have stood the test of time, techniques that have proved their worth. However technique is empty: *whatever technique we practice, whatever technique works best for us, we have to fill it. We take responsibility to make technique our own.* Ultimately this is the only way to take refuge from the storm. *And whatever the technique, it is with attitude and breath - and not with attainment - that we make the technique our own.* Making technique our own turns technique as a path into a pathless path. The path that brings us back to right here right now.

When something - in this case the idea, the concept, the metaphor of an end place and a path to get there - is not working the best strategy we have is to change it. We are asked to entertain the idea of ditching the whole getting there and path metaphor. Because there is a much more apt metaphor for the larger practice of yoga: we play games in the playground of life. And whilst on the surface the games we play differ from moment to moment, at their core they all come down to one simple choice - are we opening into, or closing away from, this present moment. In the language of yoga this choice is between a tightening and a loosening of the patterns that hold us. In the language of the Tao this choice is one of embracing or of resisting the natural flow of things.

Ultimately it is only in this present moment that we can act and produce change in our selves and by extension in the world around us. It is only right now that we can frame, explore and surrender to our experience. It is only in this present moment that we can change the game we are playing. *It is - and will only ever be - this present moment that holds the one invitation that really matters. To be right here, right now.*

Red herrings dressed up as other attractive fish. The red herrings of getting there and walking a path dress up in many guises. These guises inhabit the very mundane to the deeply philosophical, and what they have in common is that they may distract us. And part of our work and play in yoga is developing the practice of spotting our own red herrings. So here are three to get us started.

Firstly, the someone else's practice red herring: the desire for someone else's practice. The idea that once our practice looks like the person's on the mat next to us, the teacher at the front of class, or that yoga superstar we've seen on the latest branded yoga DVD, then all will be good and well; then we will be there. The someone else's practice red herring is closely related to the common manifestation of what we can call the false guru, the one who says follow my path and all will come. *Both are manifestations of a longing to be somewhere further down a path that is not there.*

Secondly, the things we snap to label as bad red herring. This red herring may show up in our yoga on the mat when we have incurred an injury. We quickly categorize the injury as something that is getting in the way of our practice. *It is something we label as bad because it will get in the way of some idea we hold as progress.* Because of our injury it's going to take us longer to get there. When we focus on the here and now, the work and play with injury as it is, is the development of our practice. All yoga practitioners who go through this process learn and grow. In more general terms - and linking it back to the Kleshas - we learn that the obstacle is the practice. We find our growth in the obstacle.

Thirdly, the red herring we will call philosophical conundrums. Typically these philosophical conundrums pop up in yoga in two forms: the who is doing the walking and the dualism versus non-dualism debates. The who is doing the walking red herring also manifests more broadly as free will versus determinism, or the question of choice. The essence of the dualism versus non-dualism debate is whether spirit and the material are one. With both these conundrums our little mind gets caught up trying to get a grip on greater mind. *Little mind gets stuck bouncing off the walls of the Idiot Box.* Both these forms can consume attention, that is our energy, to no avail. Radically simple and non-dogmatic yoga invites us to drop them from the Idiot Box and to explore the open-ended mystery of the nature of self through experiential-based practice.

We all get entangled in red herrings, and we all experience them in our own way. We also often experience that red herrings have a sort of boomerang tendency: just when we thought we disentangled they pop up again. So we continue to work through awareness and curiosity to develop discrimination. And we continue to develop our ability to see and accept what is. When we ignore, fight or story-tell around our red herrings they remain obstacles. When we observe them as they are they become doorways to depth. Now let's move on to a slightly different type of fish. Let's move on to the very attractive fish called self-development. Because one of the new traditions that emerged from yoga as it came to the West was yoga as self-development.

Self-Development? Again there is nothing wrong with self-development. However the common theme of the vast majority of methods and tools for self-development is that they work to strengthen persona. This is because mainstream self-development focuses on manifestation from ego. In contrast once our yoga kicks in we engage in a work and play that goes alot deeper than persona. If we were walking a knife-edge when it came to red herrings then now is the time to get off and pick it up. It is time to use that knife to finely fillet the very attractive fish of self-development. Then we will blow our knife up to sword size to slay the dragons of fear and laziness that guard the doorway of ego, so that we can walk through and beyond that doorway. We walk through and beyond because the yoga of the Yoga Sutras has absolutely nothing to do with self-development. *The yoga of the Yoga Sutras is the art and science of self-destruction.* To understand this we will come back to the Story Teller we introduced in the last chapter. To realise this in our being we roll out our mats and practice.

As we have seen the Story Teller is the lover of narrative. It is that part of mind that tells the stories that captivate us - the stories that lock us in and somehow define us as an individual. From this perspective the Story Teller is the lead architect in the persona construction business. And our persona is a mask - literally a false face - we put on when we go out to do our thing in the world of space, time and stuff. Persona is a mask that in a very real sense functions because from the perspective of our everyday practical experience of life we are here in the world of space, time and stuff. Therefore, and just as for ego, yoga is not about getting rid of persona: rather yoga is about moving beyond persona. Yoga invites us to explore the idea that the mask of persona is really much more like a box, a box that limits and therefore separates us.

From the perspective of yoga then, mainstream self-development is the Story Teller dressed up in its finest clothes. The Story Teller flaunting the glittering jewels of our worthy improvement goals and action plans. The Story Teller strengthening persona and building identity. *From the perspective of yoga persona is a tool for realising purpose.* And when persona is a tool for realising purpose then it follows we cannot find purpose at the level of persona. Finding purpose mandates us to move beyond the box of persona. Through yoga on our mats we grow our awareness, our ability to apply curiosity and deepen our surrender, and our yoga practice takes us beyond persona. For exploring and realising purpose we take our yoga off our mats and into our world.

Yoga as the art and science of self-destruction is yoga as spiritual practice. And make no mistake about it yoga is tough spirituality. It has to be to ride out and move beyond the storm of pleasure and pain, the storm that manifests from the Kleshas of Raga and Dvesa. It has to be as we face our ego-based fears of death - the Klesha of Abhinivesah. Because our yoga on our mats invites us to drop into the infinite flow of breath, which is the infinite flow of life. Here and now. Yoga invites us to let go of all ego props in whatever form. To let go of persona, of identity, whatever we want to call it, and ultimately to let go of the idea of our individual soul.

When we enter the world of yoga we embark on a process of change. We jump into an ocean with currents that run shallow and run deep. And when we practice we bring our focus to our own experience, to what is going down for us: the thoughts, emotions, doing and energetic patterns that are colouring our experience. Our observation of, and being with, that experience is going to take us into that ocean from shallow to deep: in its own way, at times gradually and at times in fathoms, at times with and through catharsis.

Then we come back up. We take our selves off our mat and back into the world. We re-clothe our selves in our mask of persona and go out and do our thing. Only our mask has changed. *It has become a little more porous as our realisation that a mask is just a mask deepens.* As the mask of persona becomes more porous our light inside, the light we polish through our practice, shines through a little brighter. The mask may also look and feel a little different. These differences are reflected in the feedback we receive when we go out into our world. *And ultimately, this is the litmus test that our yoga on the mat is beginning to effectuate its subtle work.* These subtle shifts in our relationship with persona are yoga made real in action.

Inner Prop: Maintain Focus

The Prop: *Focus is our ability to pay sustained attention to the work and play at hand, whatever that work may be.* And focus is a balancing act - a knife-edge that we all learn to walk. It is a balancing act between our intentional action and our non-violent abiding, our practice of letting be. Too much focus on carrying through on our actions - or rather misguided discipline - and we become rigid. Too much letting go and we end up aimlessly wandering around the well-trodden ground of our comfort zones.

Focus can also be considered a sort of balancing point of the seven props covered in this book. Focus empowers the three props we have already discussed - it really fires up the props of awareness, curiosity and surrender. And focus creates the space to allow the three props to come to unfold - it facilitates the arising of the props of purpose, mystery and creativity.

Awareness disentangles, curiosity opens our hearts, and surrender allows us to drop deeper into being. *With focus we develop our ability to sustain intentional action - both on and off our mats - from this deeper level of being.* We focus on the action for the action's sake, without expectation or attachment to the result of the action. Which is very different to intentional action with a focus on results, different to striving to impose our will upon reality.

Focus grows our ability to really pay attention to - and to zoom in on - whatever is going on down in those deeper parts of our being. *We pay attention to ever more subtle kinks in our being and to the subtle automatic doing that comes with these kinks.* Through focus we begin to really power up our practice of observation and our ability to hold our awareness in a non-violent position on whatever is going down for us. Focus empowers us as healers because it is the seeing and being with what we see - and not the act of constructing a story around that seeing - that is our healing. And focus empowers us as warriors because it is the act of staying with our edge zone that brings us to the unknown and into the territory of the warrior.

The Prop of Focus on our Mats: Our mat-based yoga is a practice of focus rather than distraction. *It is a practice of growing our ability to focus on the practice and what it brings.* Our practice is one of staying present here and now and not wandering off in time and space. And our primary practice of staying present is to bring our attention to breath.

Focusing our attention on the breath gives mind something to do. In this sense it is the master distraction that distracts mind from its habitual distractions. We bring our attention to our breathing and we bring our attention to the breath as it comes in and out of the body. And of course we wander off, so we come back to the breath again and again. This is, before and above anything else, the essence of our practice of Tapah, Svadhyaya, and Isvara-Pranidhana on our mats: our practice of discipline and dedication, of observing our selves, and of lovingly accepting our wandering and bringing our selves back to this essence. This is our practice of belly, head and heart on our mats.

And through this focus we create the space for the energy of breath - sustained by the energy of attention - to do its healing work in and of itself. This happens simply because focused attention concentrates and directs the energy of breath. As the yogis of old say *'where the attention goes, the prana flows.'*[18] So we bring this energy inside where the breath will run up against hard places. Over time, and through the repetition that focus brings, these hard places dissolve. Our attention and energy then moves on to another hard or stuck place.

Whatever our motivation for practice and whatever form that practice takes we set our focus at the start of practice. *We focus on being here and now, we focus on bringing our attention to the breath. And whatever comes up, wherever that takes us, all is good. We be with it.*

The Prop of Focus in our Worlds: The heart of our focus in our worlds is one of knowing where we are going and of knowing that this can change at any moment. We develop our ability to carry out sustained intentional action, at times in the face of considerable adversity. And we develop the ability to listen to the feedback we get as we go along. This feedback, as we tune in, will tell us when to persevere and when to change tack or ease off. This feedback supports us in walking the thin line between discipline and obstinacy.

We will get a whole lot deeper into intentional action in the next chapter when we look at taking our yoga off our mats and the warrior archetype. One more thing about focus before we move on: when focus feels like work that is because it is. It is a sort of work that seems to be inherently fulfilling because although focus is work, it is also play. Just ask anyone who has focused to move towards mastery of something for a sustained period of time.

5. Taking Yoga Off Our Mats

Our practice on our mats prepares us for taking our yoga into our worlds. Prepares us for embodying the attitude of the warrior, for stepping into the unknown, for taking a risk and exposing our selves to some sort of loss. In our worlds we explore and manifest purpose.

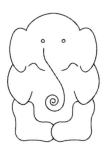

The Yoga of the Bhagavad Gita

Our warrior's choice. In Chapter Two we touched on the Bhagavad Gita when we looked at Our Big Shift. We discussed how the Bhagavad Gita recounts a conversation between the warrior Arjuna and his charioteer Sri Krishna. This conversation, which is part of the larger narrative the Mahabharata, takes place just before Arjuna, his brothers, and their armies take to the battlefield. We looked at the essence of that conversation - the instruction that Krishna gives Arjuna in yoga. Now we will dig a little deeper into that instruction, a little deeper into what is traditionally brought and taught as three paths of yoga. Then we will link that up to our practices of yoga on the mat and look at the radical and simple message that is behind the idea of paths.

The Bhagavad Gita is broadly considered to present yoga for every man and woman whatever their life circumstances. It presents the yoga of being out in the world: that is where Arjuna is, out in the world doing his thing. Although when the conversation of the Bhagavad Gita takes place we can more accurately say that Arjuna is not doing his thing: he has hit a wall of indecision and needs a little help. The help he receives is the instruction from Krishna. The first instruction that Krishna gives Arjuna is in Karma yoga. Karma yoga is - like our practice of Tapah on our mats - the yoga of action. Karma yoga is the yoga of doing rooted in our belly. And, just like Tapah, it is most importantly the carrying out of action - of doing our work - without attachment to the results. Or, to use another common terminology, Karma yoga is the yoga of selfless service, and to be very clear Karma yoga is not about detachment or indifference. *Just like our practice of Tapah on our mat, the heart of Karma yoga is passionate involvement in what we are doing in this moment. It is an attitude of, the journey is the reward.*

The second yoga that Krishna instructs is Jnana yoga, the yoga of knowledge, of knowledge as wisdom from experience. Jnana yoga is - just like our practice of Svadhyaya on our mats - the yoga of using intention and discrimination to explore the nature of self. Through that exploration of self we gain wisdom and understanding not only about our selves but also about the larger reality in which we are embedded. Jnana yoga is often thought of as yoga for the renunciant, yoga for those who have retreated from the world: the meditator hidden away in the cave; the monk in the monastery and; the spiritual seeker in the Ashram. *However in the context of the Bhagavad Gita Krishna instructs Arjuna in Jnana Yoga so that he can use it in his world, on his battlefield, to do his work.* That is where he has to apply his discrimination in action and this is something that holds true for all of us as we live our lives.

The third yoga that Krishna instructs is Bhakti yoga - the yoga of devotion and in particular, in the context of the Bhagavad Gita, devotion to Krishna. Krishna, like many in the Indian pantheon of deities, is a playful fellow and not one to pass up an opportunity to say: devote all to me. Krishna, more pertinently though, is one of the incarnations of the Hindu god Vishnu and Vishnu represents, or is a metaphor for, the all-pervading essence of the universe. *In this sense the practice of Bhakti yoga is a practice of surrendering to this essence, of moving towards and merging with this essence.* The essence of Bhakti is in the surrendering and not in how we frame or label that essence: Bhakti yoga is the surrendering, and opening our hearts, to what is. This is analogous to the practice of Isvara-Pranidhana on our mat.

Just like the Yoga Sutras, the Bhagavad Gita is a text of great depth with many ways of framing its message. Traditionally - that is, in the context of tradition - the most common way of framing that message is one that is essentially reductionist. It is reductionist because the instruction that

Krishna gives in yoga is broken down and brought to us as three paths of yoga: the first path being the path of selfless action, or the spiritual pillar of service; the second being the path of wisdom, or the spiritual pillar of mindfulness; and the third being the path of devotion, or the spiritual pillar of gratitude. Traditions then often present us with a choice between paths of yoga. The rationale usually given for this reduction is that we are all different and different paths suit people with different dispositions. This reduction however, implies that Arjuna's choice, and by extension our choice, and responsibility is reduced to choosing and walking a path.

Although the three paths of yoga is the way the message of the Bhagavad Gita is commonly brought to us there is - as we touched on early in Chapter Two - a much more powerful message lying behind the text. Given all the ground we have covered since Chapter Two we now know this. We know this because we know that in yoga reductionism is just a tool: a tool to support us in moving beyond separation to connection. We know this because we know that our simple framework of the anatomy and yogas of belly, head and heart is just a framework. It is a framework we use to explore and ultimately let go of as our practices of yoga on the mat become one, just as the spiritual pillars of service, mindfulness and gratitude merge into one. And we know this because we know that paths are just another red herring that the world of separation throws our way to distract our attention away from our work at hand. It is time to get radical again, time to go back to the roots, and it is time to get simple.

The radically simple message of the Bhagavad Gita is one of holistic agency. It is a message of whole being empowerment, of taking and growing our response-ability. Because what Krishna is saying to Arjuna is essentially: *You are not who or what you think you are. You are however here in this big interconnected world and you're always playing your part, you are always doing something. Each moment contains a requirement to action. Use your belly, your head and your heart and act: act with intelligence and act through love.*

Then Krishna passes the ball to Arjuna saying *you choose*, and *it is by taking his decision and making his move that Arjuna becomes a yogic warrior.* Arjuna makes his move from a position of wisdom and with an open heart, and in doing so embodies the message of the Bhagavad Gita as awakened realisation of purpose. Arjuna steps up to playing his part in the whole. *For our yoga this means that to awaken we look inside - we practice on our mats - and to make that awakening real we take our selves off the mat and into the world.* This is the warrior's choice that we all face. The radical simplicity of this choice becomes a little clearer when we look at the Bhagavad Gita from another perspective: when we examine the Bhagavad Gita as myth.

The prop of myth. Besides its place in the Mahabharata the Bhagavad Gita is also often taken to be a text in its own right. It is a spiritual text that uses a story in the world outside to rub up against the inexplicable of the world inside. To do this the Bhagavad Gita uses the prop of myth, which is a very powerful prop. *When we look at the text in this way the Bhagavad Gita is a metaphor: Arjuna's struggle may be on the battlefield but the struggle the Gita speaks to as myth is our own struggle.* From this perspective both Arjuna and Krishna are placeholders. Arjuna is the placeholder for every man and every woman, for each of us. Arjuna is the placeholder for our individual consciousness, for the one who acts and produces effect in the world. Krishna is the placeholder for any God or source of power, external or internal. Krishna is the placeholder for universal consciousness that is the source of our courage to open our minds and hearts and to act accordingly.

Early on in her book *A Short History of Myth*[19], the scholar, author and commentator Karen Armstrong lays out five important points about myth in general. We will look at these five points in the context of the Bhagavad Gita. The first point that Armstrong makes is that myth *"is nearly always rooted in the experience of death and the fear of extinction."* Arjuna's fear of extinction is real, both for himself and for his loved ones facing each other across the battlefield. Battle is about to be waged and with battle come death and destruction. *In the Bhagavad Gita Arjuna's courage is rooted in another experience of death that, although less tangible, is just as real.* Arjuna finds courage in the death of a belief, the belief of separation - death of a belief that stems from Arjuna's realisation of Krishna's message that all is One. The fear of death, both of our ego and our physical body, is something we all have and that we all face sooner or later. Our practice of yoga invites us all to let go of the belief of separation, and it is through facing the fears this brings that we find courage.

The second point that Armstrong makes is that *"mythology is usually inseparable from ritual,"* and the yoga of the Bhagavad Gita is steeped in ritual. The yoga of the Bhagavad Gita is yoga with strong bonds to traditions that use tools such as paths, ethics, and ritual to offer us structure and sanctuary. In the context of the Bhagavad Gita it is Bhakti yoga in particular that is inseparable from the tool of ritual. Bhakti yoga is the yoga of devotion given structure and offering sanctuary through ritual such as puja, fire ceremony and the chanting of the names of various aspects of the One. *All these rituals are designed to open our hearts to the One, to love, and when we engage in these rituals with purity of intention we both surrender to the power of, and transcend, the form of the ritual.*

Thirdly Armstrong states that *"the most powerful myths are often about extremity; they force us to go beyond our experience."* Myth invites us to take a step into the unknown, and the conversation between Arjuna and Krishna takes place exactly when Arjuna finds himself at the cusp of the unknown. It takes place when Arjuna finds himself in a position of extremity about to go to battle. The invitation Krishna offers Arjuna to move on and into the new plays out at different levels. It plays out at the very practical level of the battlefield and it plays out at the level of worldviews - an invitation to shift from separation to connection. And it plays out for Arjuna at the level of heart, of surrender to what is, to devoting his actions to the good of all. *This broad all-encompassing invitation is one we all face, albeit that for many of us our step into the new is one we take from a position of less extremity than Arjuna.*

When it comes to action the instructions of yoga that Krishna gives Arjuna are in essence teachings in living. These teachings are for Arjuna in the situation of extremity he finds himself in and for all of us wherever we find our selves. Just as, and perhaps more familiarly, the teachings of the Buddha in right living are known as Dharma, Krishna's instructions can be framed as Dharma teachings. Which brings us on to the fourth point made by Armstrong: *"mythology puts us in the correct spiritual or psychological posture for right action, in this world or the next."* In the context of the myth of the Bhagavad Gita Dharma has a second meaning: Arjuna's duty as warrior. Krishna's message serves to remind Arjuna of his duty - his purpose - as a warrior. A duty to follow through with action on what his lifelong training has prepared him for. *Action taken for the good of all, and that is taken from and grounded within spirit.* Which brings us on to the last point that Armstrong makes.

Armstrong's fifth and final point is that *"all mythology speaks of another plane that exists alongside our own world, and that in some sense supports it."* This point, as far as the teachings of the Bhagavad Gita for a world of connection are concerned, may not go quite far enough. Because in the worldview of the yogis of old that other plane, the plane of spirit, does not exist alongside our common perception to our world: *it is intimately interconnected with, and ultimately, is our world. Spirit does not only support our world in some sense; that support comes in and of itself.*

When we look at the Bhagavad Gita through the perspective of myth then the text is not only instruction in yoga. The Bhagavad Gita serves to help us make sense of the world we find our selves in, the world as one big interconnected thing. And it serves to support us in how to live our lives, it supports us in the struggle we all face with, and between, two forces. One force is the opening up to the new, to the unlimited potential of this present moment. The other force is the closing in to our past. This is a struggle we can also frame as one between a benevolent and a malevolent force, the struggle that perhaps is one of the defining characteristics of our human condition. This struggle becomes yoga when we awaken to the potential for radical - that is, deep rooted - change in our own lifetime. This is the change that is founded in the experiences of our journey into connection within. We realise - very literally, make real - this change when we take the wisdom of belly, head and heart off our mats and into our world. This change is grounded in exploration of purpose.

Explore purpose. Yoga is a practice for life - both in the sense of our life as a whole and in the sense of a lifelong practice. It is a practice that serves us on and off our mats and that grows with us as we grow. This is the same as saying that our work and play with the inner props of yoga - our attitude skills - is one that never ends. This work and play is a process of mastery. Just like our practice of yoga Asana, over time we become more skilful and over time new space opens up for our work and play. This is the power and beauty of yoga as a system for personal empowerment. And when it comes to purpose the important thing is this: in yoga there is no quick fix to finding purpose. *In yoga we explore purpose and we act to realise purpose with the wisdom of that exploration wherever we are right now.* Purpose is not fixed; it deepens, morphs, and shifts as we do.

Purpose in yoga is birthed from that space inside. This space also births us our sense of joy, of peace and that is our power. Our yoga practice on our mats serves in essence to connect us with - and to strengthen that connection with - that space inside. This is the sweetest fruit of our practice. This is the sweet fruit that comes in and of it self as we loosen our selves from the grip of the Kleshas. And as this connection is strengthened our persona - that mask we put on to go out and do our thing - becomes infused with the energy of that space inside.

The biggest challenge many of us face is in allowing this energy inside to shine through our persona. In this, and in our modern world, it may at times seem as if all the cards are stacked against us. To empower us in this we take the perspective of our practice of yoga on our mats as warrior practice. It is our practice that grows our ability to connect with, and act from, spirit, from that space inside. It is our practice that grows the conditions that allow spirit to manifest through persona outside of our allocated practice times. This allowing comes from intentional action manifested with courage and compassion in our hearts. So let's dive a little deeper into yoga as a warrior practice.

The Warrior Archetype

Yoga as warrior practice. The warrior is one of the most powerful archetypes in traditions East and West, and down through the ages, and the warrior archetype is integral to yoga. Many of us who practice yoga on our mats are familiar with the warrior postures: a sequence of postures named after, and illustrating, a certain story in Indian mythology. And of course there is the warrior Arjuna the troubled hero of the Bhagavad Gita: Arjuna who, paralysed by indecision, sits down before battle to ask questions and receive instruction in yoga from Krishna. In this section we will look at the metaphor of the warrior in yoga. In particular we will look at a number of aspects that define the warrior in the context of our yoga or, in other words, how the warrior archetype meshes with the mat-based yoga so popular in the West today.[20]

The first key point with respect to defining the warrior, and that is relevant in the context of our yoga, is practice. When we look at any warrior tradition - such as the Samurai of Japan, the warriors of the Sheik faith or the native Indians of the Americas - then the practice of one or more warrior arts is an essential and common element across all traditions. This practice may be one that we conventionally think of as a warrior art such as swordsmanship or a mind-body practice like Tai Chi, or it may be something we think of as more esoteric such as entering and exploring the dream world. Arjuna practiced many warrior arts and his core practice was archery. Whilst the form of the practice differs across the different cultures all warrior practices are a vehicle for developing self-mastery: through practice the warrior grows their understanding of self and their ability to intentionally direct self in action.

As modern yogis when we frame our mat-based practice as our warrior art then our mat-based practice is our training ground for developing self-mastery. Through our yoga practice we develop self-mastery in the form of strength and flexibility: strength and flexibility of body, mind and spirit; flexibility of doing and of being; and flexibility in seeing, in our choice of perspective on reality. We develop self-mastery through the recognition and disentanglement from patterns: patterns that no longer serve us and are draining our energy. Our self-mastery through yoga on our mats is a vehicle for developing the skills of focus, discipline and intention, and for growing our ability to be with, and surrender to, whatever is going down for us right here, right now.

All warrior traditions recognize that self-mastery is a process that never ends. For the warrior their practice is an ongoing invitation to expand their experience and use of self. This is exactly the invitation given to us by our yoga practice once we disentangle our selves from the temptation of yoga as a path with a destination, from yoga as achievement. This is the invitation we open to when we practice yoga in a way that is radical and simple. For the warrior who has realised that self-mastery is ongoing this brings the obligation to step into the unknown: it is in the unknown that new knowledge of self is to be found, and in the unknown where new use of self is to be learned. In this respect too, and for the yogi as warrior, our mat-based practice is our training ground since our yoga on our mats brings us time and time again to a point where we have never been before. Our practice brings us to a point where we are invited to acknowledge and engage with the uniqueness of each and every present moment: a point where we are invited to step into the new. Which is exactly the invitation we engage with when we take our yoga off our mats into our worlds. This brings us on to the second key point that defines the warrior and that is relevant to our yoga.

The second key point in defining a warrior is that their practice is not only a vehicle for growing self-mastery: it is through their practice that the warrior grows their understanding of the world they find their self in. The warriors grows their understanding both in the allocated time for practicing their warrior art and as the attitude of the warrior infuses the way they are and act in their world. This understanding, just like the process of self-mastery, is one they build and develop with the explicit recognition that getting there is not an option: all warrior traditions pay deep respect to the mysterious nature of reality.

This aspect of the warrior is analogous to the non-dogmatic approach when we practice yoga in a way that is both radical and simple. As we saw right back in Chapter One it is the wisdom we gain through the experience of practice that informs our worldview. Or framing this in terms of the three big questions we looked at in Chapter One it is our exploration of the *'who am I?'* question that feeds the *'what is this world I find myself in?'* question. Very specifically our yoga - and this holds true for the warrior arts in all traditions - expands our perspective on the first and then the second of these questions by loosening us from the grip of ego. This brings us on to the third and last point we will cover here: a point that is directly related to that third big question we covered in Chapter One, *'what to do?'*

The third key point is that the warrior steps - as and when required - into the unknown to act with intention and produce effect on their world. This point builds on the previous two: analogous to the fourth point we explored when we looked at myth, for the warrior the practice of their warrior art prepares them for right action. Their practice builds strength and flexibility in their psychosomatic architecture and builds awareness and understanding of the world around them. So that when they make their move into the unknown they are able to respond with maximum effect in each moment as it unfolds. When the warrior moves from their training ground to their battleground they make their move into the unknown in the full knowledge that they may or may not realise the effect they intend. When they step into the unknown they take a purposeful risk and by taking this step the warrior faces fear and gains courage and knowledge. These three points capture the essence of the metaphor of yoga as a warrior art, and together with yoga as a practice for loosening from pattern, illustrate the central idea of this book of yoga as a personal empowerment technology. This is all tied together in the illustration below.

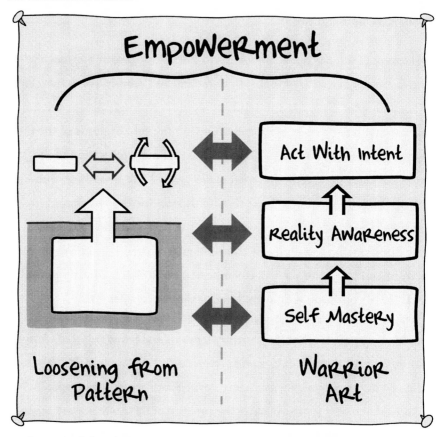

At the end of the Bhagavad Gita Arjuna, having receiving instruction from Krishna, sets his intent and purpose. Arjuna the warrior takes his risk; he picks up his arms and goes to battle. We have seen that in the metaphor of yoga as a warrior art our mat-based practice is our training ground for developing self-mastery and growing our understanding of reality. Our mat-based practice is also - in a very real sense - our battleground as warriors. It is our battleground because on our mats we are up against the forces of habit, the forces of pattern that pull us back to our familiar ways of engagement with each moment. These habitual ways of engagement are, as we have seen, characterised by the pull of our likes and dislikes, by our ego's games and its fear of death, and that by being there and then, rather than here and now. As warriors on our mats the arms we take with us to our battles are not the sword or the bow and arrow: ultimately all we have is method - our relationship with breath - and our attitude skills. It is by facing our battles on our mats that we set in motion the realisation of broader personal transformation.

Realisation. Yoga is a process of transformation, of personal change. Yoga brings change in our internal architecture and in our outward action - when our wisdom from experience infuses what we do and how we do it. This transformation is actualised in the embodiment of our wisdom of belly, head and heart when we go out and be and do in our worlds to make it real.

This realisation is the tough part for many of us. Just like our practice of loosening from pattern on our mats, realisation is where the rubber hits the road. One of the reasons we find it tough is because many of us get entangled in a pattern where we put a little box around our practice time - our weekly trip to class or our daily practice at home. Outside of this box we get back to doing our thing in our habitual ways. However when we do not move to realise outwards, if our behaviours do not shift and change, then yoga as a system for personal empowerment is not going to fly.

Whilst we each have to do our own work and play when it comes to realisation, the metaphor of yoga as a warrior practice provides a framework for realisation. It provides a useful map to support us in our work and play. *This map begins with recognition and very specifically the recognition that the patterns that colour our habitual experience on our mats are exactly the patterns that colour our experience in our worlds.* Our own work and play means we each recognise our own signposts for the patterns that are most manifest in our own experience: patterns like stress, a hunkering for external recognition, of end-gaming, and the patterns of fear and laziness. The pressure cooker of our practice time grows our awareness - and through awareness our recognition - of these patterns. These patterns are not at all interested in any arbitrary line that we draw between our practice time and the rest of our lives.

Our map for realisation moves on from recognition to intention and then to action aligned with that intention. Formulating intention and carrying through on intentional action is something we all practice on our mats. And whatever else we do on our mats we all practice this in a number of ways. Firstly we do this through growing our ability to work and play on our mats in a way that is safe. In this way we minimise the possibility of incurring injury or distress to our selves - both acute and chronic, and to the physical body as well as mentally, emotionally, and energetically. The second way we do this is through growing our ability to practice in a way that is functional whatever our motivations for practice: whether we practice to relax, practice with a focus on a certain area of our physical body - an area where we may have a poor connection, a lack of strength or a tightness - or practice to explore our relationship with breath. Or simply when we practice for the sake of practice. Thirdly, and when we practice yoga in a way that is radical and simple, we grow our ability to hold our attention on our attitude to practice.

Realisation off our mats necessitates taking the skills of intentional action to our behaviours off our mats. We do this when it comes to loosening our selves from the patterns that are most manifest in our experience, and we do this when it comes to creating something new: something more aligned with our experience of connection inside. In both cases we essentially set an intention and act to do something different. And to do something different is to resist the temptation of the familiar. So - for example - we step back from stress rather than moving deeper into entanglement. Or we refocus on the process here and now rather than the results we hope to achieve in our work. And we refocus on the here and now to disentangle our selves from the patterns of fear and laziness.

When it comes to creating something new, and most relevantly in the context of our yoga and our big shift, then a powerful prop is inspiration. Because when we look around we see people who are standing up and acting from the belief that a better world is possible. This is a world free of the striving, imbalance and dis-ease we see today. These are the people who are stepping outside of the values and structures of the old and doing something different, and who are working to create a world where we value flow, balance and harmony. *The people who are standing up are the ones who are reclaiming their agency, their ability to act and produce effect in the world from a specific perspective.*

These are the ones who have realised only we can let go of a belief that holds us. They embody the truth that only we can transform our common experience of connection from an intellectual concept - from just another dogma - into a realisation, into an empowered belief that infuses what we do and how we do it. They embody the truth that no one else can do this for us, that ultimately this is work and play we each do on our own. And they are doing this in each and every area of our communal lives. So we look around, each from our own perspective, and we find our inspiration. Wherever we find our selves, and whatever our passions, we can find inspiration - there are no hard and fast rules here and no one size fits all.

So to link back up to something we covered right back at the start of Chapter One: yoga wakes us up and yoga wakes us up in a way that is the more we all want. So yoga does not just wake us up in a dry compartmentalised way that is confined to our time on our mats. *We want to wake up in a way that effects change in our selves, in our lives and in our worlds.* We want to wake up in a way that facilitates manifesting different behaviours: behaving with a different attitude and acting from awareness. Yoga wakes us up to playing our part in creating the new in whatever way fits with where we are. Our map for realizing our waking up is shown in the illustration below which also includes the steps of navigation and feedback.

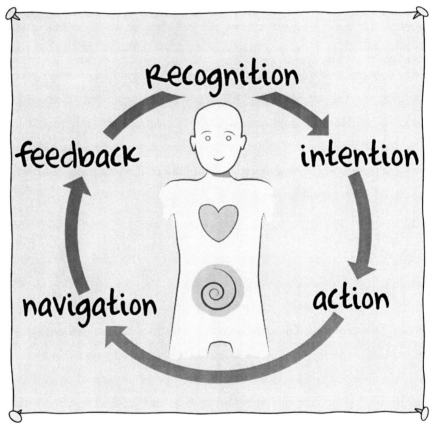

Navigation and feedback follow our action because when we do something different we step into the new, we step into the unknown. And when we step into the unknown we do not know what is going to happen. This is part and parcel of doing something different. Stuff is going to happen that we did not expect, that we could not foresee. So we ease off on expectation, we remain flexible and open to feedback, and we grow our ability to navigate the complexity of the unknown. In this way our intentional action in our world is much more akin to a directional thrust than a specific goal or objective. It is the purpose behind the action that is key, not the exact form of its manifestation as a specific goal.

Our practices of yoga for belly, head and heart feed beautifully and seamlessly into our map for realisation in our worlds. These practices support each of us in finding the right balance between discipline and fluidity in perception and action that facilitate sustainable realisation. Through our practice of Tapah, or Karma yoga, we grow our ability to act for the sake of the action. We grow discipline in and dedication to our actions. We ease off expectation and specifically we ease off our attachment to manifestation of our actions in specific form. Through our practice of Svadhyaya we grow our ability to see things as they are, both when it comes to recognition of the old and when we step into the new. And we grow our ability to shift our perspective as we integrate the wisdom of our current experience into our internal architecture. Through our practice of Isvara-Pranidhana, or Bhakti, we grow compassion and courage in our hearts. This courage grows - and grows with - our responsibility in the face of the never-ending magic of each present moment.

Building and taking courage. Realisation in our worlds rests above all else on, and brings with it, courage. It takes courage to break with the illusion of destiny imposed upon us by our entanglement in pattern. Initiating and following through with skill in action that competes with what seems to be our fate brings courage.[21] And courage, in yoga as life, really does live up to the old classroom riddle of what came first, the chicken or the egg. On one side of this riddle as metaphor our training ground as warriors on our mats provides a safe - or at least relatively safe - environment for exploring the new. We explore making subtle changes in how we embody each posture; we explore shifting the focus of our attention; and we play with our perspective in our relationship with breath. In this sense our yoga on our mats is training ground for breaking with pattern and building courage in very tangible ways.

In a less tangible way - but still on the same side of the chicken and egg metaphor - our practices of yoga on our mats build courage in and of themselves. *As long as we maintain our focus on, and grow our alignment with, the simple practices of belly, head and heart.* When we practice with this focus we grow connection with our deep source of strength and courage, with that same source that gifts us peace and joy, happiness and purpose. This is the space inside that in the world of connection we can call spirit; raw spirit unboxed by plays of our ego minds. It is spirit abiding in our ignorance of our nature and infusing all aspects of our being. Our practice on our mats therefore builds courage both in very tangible and less tangible ways, and both ways support us when we explore the new off our mats.

Moving to the other side of the chicken and egg metaphor: *as we have seen, when we take our yoga off our mats there is always a step to take. This is a step we ultimately take alone and outside the training ground of our mats.* It is a step we take in the face of fear and it is in the act of taking that step that we take courage. Or perhaps better said, take back the courage that is our birthright. *In other words we do the thing we fear and the courage comes afterwards.* So on this side of the metaphor we take courage by acknowledging and acting in the face of our fears.

It is with courage that we start to embody yoga as a system for personal empowerment outside of our allocated practice times. It is with courage that we take the wisdom we gain from our practice off our mats and out into our worlds. It is with courage that we start to embody our worldview as warriors of the new in the way we are, and in what and how we do, in our lives as a whole. In short: it is with courage that the opportunity arises for, and we open up to the invitation of, changing direction.

At some point or other we take that opportunity and at other times the opportunity takes us. At yet other times it may not be at all clear who or what is doing the taking. The key is this: yoga as a warrior art informs our actions. We act in the knowledge that we are under no obligation to continue to be held by beliefs we have grown out of, no obligation to hold on to beliefs that are no longer useful. Above all we act under the obligation to act - this is the blessing and burden of yoga as a warrior art, of yoga as skill in action. This is the blessing and burden of Krishna's parting shot to Arjuna that in essence is: *'now that you have received the instruction of yoga, act and devote all to me.'*

This brings us on to a final - and essential - point with respect to the warrior archetype and yoga as a warrior art: devotion. Devotion plays a central role in all warrior traditions, although this devotion takes many forms: devotion to a master, to a guru, to a god or gods of various forms. *What warriors in all traditions have in common is devotion to the purpose behind their art: a dedication to embracing and exploring through action the mystery of the world we find our selves in.* For the yogi, who finds him or herself in the midst of the whole big interconnected whatever-you-want-to-call-it, dedication to the purpose behind our yoga as warrior art is dedication to the One manifesting now from moment to moment. This is the dedication to building and taking courage for action for the good of all. It is the dedication to grounding within - and acting from - spirit as love that is yoga made real in action.

Inner Prop: Explore Purpose

The Prop: This prop is emphatically one of exploring, and it runs so against the grain of our conditioning in our modern world that a point made earlier is worth repeating here: for the yogi there is no quick fix to finding purpose. *Rather than finding purpose for our persona, our work and play in yoga is much more akin to allowing purpose to manifest through persona.* This manifestation arises from our connection with that space that is beyond our ego-self; it arises from beyond our little mind.

Whilst our manifestation of purpose will morph and shift as we strengthen this connection, *this is a manifestation that does not wait on time.* There is no getting there - we are always manifesting here and now, from wherever we are and whatever the depth and strength of our connection. It is in this sense that our relationship with purpose is one of exploration. It is an exploration that has no final destination, one that unfolds within and before us, as we act on our mats and in our worlds.

The Prop of Purpose on our Mats: **Our practice of yoga on our mats is a practice of exploring rather than finding.** It is an invitation in - at least - two very specific ways to explore purpose. Firstly an invitation to explore what is the right way for us to practice. Accepting this invitation requires courage: the courage we build through the wisdom from experience in practice, and the courage we take as we grow responsibility for our practice. Because when we practice we use all sorts of techniques and tools. Techniques and tools, that however they were transmitted in the past, are now overwhelmingly transmitted in the modern class environment. And when it comes to the modern class environment the general rule is the more the merrier.

The growth of modern class-based yoga teaching has been accompanied by standardisation. In particular standardisation - or rather competing forms, styles or brands of standardisation - in the right way to practice Asana. Like all things in yoga this is neither good nor bad; for most of us it serves a very useful purpose as we learn the ropes. At some point our focus begins to shift. This is a shift from doing our practice right to the right practice for us between and within any form of mat-based yoga we may be practicing.

At some point yoga invites us to make our practice our own. Which for many in yoga means to start practicing at home where we are away from the distractions of the class environment, away from the constant stream of technical instruction and the self-imposed pressures to conform in physical Asana and movement. When we practice alone we can create an environment where we focus on making breath primary in our practice and in particular we can focus on surrendering into breath. In this environment we grow our response-ability, our ability to respond, in increasingly subtle ways to the feedback from our experience. We grow our ability to connect with and experience the mysterious infinite inside. Which brings us on to the second invitation when it comes to exploring purpose on our mats.

When we take the perspective of the yoga of the Bhagavad Gita, the perspective of yoga as a warrior art, the primary purpose of practice is one of exploring what it means to live within and from spirit. This is another way of looking at the essence of Krishna's message to Arjuna. *So from this perspective our practice on our mats is a practice of embodiment from spirit.* It is a practice of embodiment within and from the mystery of breath, the mystery of life.

The Prop of Purpose in our Worlds: Exploring purpose in our worlds means taking purposeful risks. This is something each of us learns in our own way. Risk means very simply that we expose our selves to some sort of loss through our actions.[22] We take a risk that is appropriate in that it takes us out of our comfort zone and into our edge zone. It takes us into a space where we allow, and allow our selves to allow, something new to happen. And this risk is appropriate in that we weigh that loss against the purpose of our actions. Purpose that over times loosens from and then - metaphorically speaking - moves behind our mask of persona.

From each step in purposeful risk-taking we receive our feedback and we learn. Learning that flows when we look at our feedback from a position of non-violence. Which for many of us means dropping the tendency to blame our selves, others, or circumstances for what we may jump to label as failure in our actions. With this dropping we shift towards embodying the attitude of the warrior - we move beyond the victim trap in its many manifestations.

Very specifically it means dropping our tendency to use the yogi's concept of Karma as a whip for self-flagellation. We shift to seeing Karma as the universe's feedback mechanism: the One talking to itself in balance and flow. We shift to picking our selves back up when we fall and taking a new step. This is a shift towards acting from and within spirit. *When we live in spirit, although it may look to some on the outside that nothing much has changed, in essence we act in a way that is radically different.*

6. Balance and Flow

Behind our hardened worldview of space and time reality manifests in balance and flow. To engage in this reality through our work and play on and off our mats is to get spiritual. Embracing the mystery that is beyond knowing mind deepens this engagement.

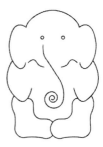

The Way Things Are

Worldview shift. When our yoga starts to kick in, when our yoga does what it says on the box, our explorations inside and out in our world take us deeper into the mystery of self. The deeper we journey the more we are able to see those boundaries between inside and out for what they are: constructs of our personal and collective minds, and demarcations valid at the level of the gross material. At one level our yoga on our mats and in our worlds teaches us that some of these boundaries are functional whereas others are not, or at least no longer, so. We all experience our own grey area between the functional and the dysfunctional; at this level it is our exploration of this grey area that gifts us our opportunities for freedom and empowerment. *At another level our seeing alone brings freedom because with our seeing the hardness of these boundaries softens, crumbles, and dissolves, and our sense of mystery seeps from inside to out.* We are invited to entertain the idea that our worldview of a play of separate things on a stage of space and time may not be as solid as we thought.

Our modern culture programmes and pushes us to accept without questioning this worldview of separate things on a stage of space and time as reality. This worldview has always had, and will always have, a place simply because at a very practical level it works: on the whole it seems to mesh pretty well with the information we receive from our senses and it serves us as we go about and do stuff. This is the worldview embraced and explored by mainstream Western science. Science, for a long time, focused on breaking things down into pieces and studying those pieces to define laws that govern the relationship between them. Science now has laws for the very large, the very small, and everything in between. With the scientific underpinning of the worldview of separate objects these laws are given the role of kings and queens on the stage of life; these laws determine how the play on the stage pans out and the basic dimensions of this stage are space and time.

In step with the ascension of modern science this worldview has become omnipotent; it has crowded out all others. *This worldview has pushed all other perspectives on reality out to the wastelands in the margins of our individual and collective being.* Over the years necessity, logic, ridicule, in fact any strategy available, have all been used so that this perspective on reality now permeates every aspect of our lives. Independently of the specifics of which worldview dominates, a lack of competing worldviews is a sign of an unhealthy world. And it is our specific dominant worldview that brings with it our entanglement in the efficiency machine where we focus on solving problems, on dealing with stuff and moving on. It is our specific worldview of separation that has led to neglect of the planet, community and self. Behind our dominant worldview lies an assumption: the assumption that we can somehow extract our selves from reality and observe it. The observer and the observed are separate and by extension the observer can step back and command and control the observed. In short we have succumbed to the temptation to believe that we were in control; that we could play God outside the whole. And in this process we have lost a lot. *Simply because essence, richness and intelligence are in relationship - they are in the whole.*

Science however has an interesting, or perhaps a dirty, little secret. This is a little secret that the foot soldiers of science and its technology applications keep pushing under the carpet and one about which the leading lights of science are quite open: science cannot really get a grasp on space and time. Scientists can draw up ways of measuring and of describing space and time, but measuring and describing are not the same as explaining. And where there is no explanation the mystery begins.

Balance and flow. The worldview from the ancient East is a very different one to that of the play of separate objects on a stage of space and time. *The best metaphor for the worldview from the East is one of the One at play.* This is the core of the Vedic texts of old that form the basis for yoga philosophy and practices. This is the core that is found in the more mythological side of the yoga literature: a pantheon of Gods representing different aspects of the One engaged in timeless play. Play, incidentally, that just like in the ancient Greek mythology of the West consists mainly of the struggles of war and of the pleasures of lovemaking. The One at play is also the core of the Taoist worldview: the mysterious Tao that permeates everything and that manifests in the ten thousand things.

When the best metaphor we have for the One is some sort of energy, and the simplest division of one is into two, then the best metaphor we have for two is two energies. So with the worldview of the One at play come the stories of a split of the One into two energies. This split into two energies is the basic metaphor or framework underlying the philosophy and the practices of the yoga traditions and those of the Taoist arts. Now the basic qualities of energy are balance and flow. Therefore, with the worldview of the ancient East, one of the key ideas we are invited to entertain is this: when it is useful to divide reality, to apply a basic reductionism, then balance and flow are the fundamental characteristics of the world we find ourselves in and part of. This idea is the key and not the metaphor for this division.

In the Hatha yoga traditions the metaphor for this split into two energies is that of Shiva and Shakti. In more mythological language this is framed as life playing out through the dance of Shiva and Shakti. Where Shiva represents pure consciousness, whatever that may be, or in terms of energy Shiva represents stillness as potential. Shakti represents manifestation or the movement of energy as realisation. The essence of the Hatha Yoga practices is an exploration of the dance between and union of these two experiences of energy. *In the Tantra yoga traditions some schools use another metaphor - that of expanding and contracting energy.* The metaphor is one of opening and closing and these schools focus practice on the exploration of opening and closing: exploring our experience of opening and closing from an ever-greater sense of self. In particular they focus on the practice of surrendering to the opening - of devotion to the opening - to negate our inborn and inbred tendencies of closing. *In Taoism the metaphor for the basic split of the One into two is that of Yin and Yang energies.* Where Yin is passive or non-doing, and Yang is active or doing. The essence of Taoist arts such as Tai Chi is the exploration of balance and flow between doing and non-doing.

However we frame these two energies the key thing is that both are always present and contained within each other. One perspective we can take on our practice of yoga on our mat and taking our yoga off the mat and into our world is that we can see these energies in terms of coming home and going out. When we go out into our world we need the energy of impetus and direction otherwise we stagnate. And then things become static and flow stops. Too much impetus out into the world and the material world of things becomes our reality and we lose the less tangible things in life. We lose connection with spirit, lose connection with life force. So whilst going out we need the energy of coming home, we need warmth and receptivity. And when coming home we need the seed of going out. Without this seed, with only warmth and receptivity we risk clinging to, to holding on and becoming stuck. And again flow stops. *So wherever we are right now these two energies play together in evolution and this play is balance and flow in action.*

Let's return one more time to our discussion of East meets West and the message of modern science. Many voices in mainstream or traditional science succumb to the temptation to say give us a few more years and we will figure it all out. Our knowing minds will always be tempted to grasp for the carrot of completion. However, what modern science invites us to entertain is that the worldview of the ancient East - the metaphor of the One at play - may just be a little closer to the indescribable reality that is. Or put another way it may just be so that the world of space and time is manifested from a much more mysterious world characterised by balance and flow, as shown below.

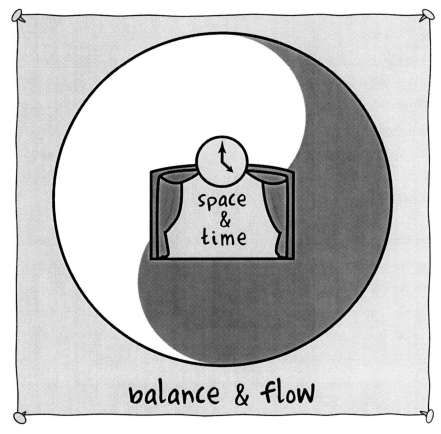

This is in a very real sense the reality that we acquaint our selves with through yoga. This is also the more we all want from our yoga: an ever deeper connection with our source of happiness, of freedom and of purpose. This more is a yearning for a merging with the energy of the One, with the energy of the Gods. We desire to realise our part, our wholeness, in the One at play.

One last and essential thing about balance and flow: both balance and flow are dynamic. For flow this is self-evident: when it is not flowing, when it is static or stuck, then it is not flow. And whilst balance may appear static, it too is dynamic: the moment we try to fix something in balance - when we try to snap it to static - then it shifts. Balance moves from moment to moment. This is one thing we all learn from the balancing poses such as headstand or tree pose in Asana practice.

Embrace mystery. At a very practical level yoga is a set of tools for living in harmony with the world. Or to take this one step further: yoga is living in harmony with the world. This living in harmony with the world comes from rubbing up really close to reality, from merging with the bigger picture, from becoming one with life. Life that is - in the Eastern worldview - characterised by balance and flow. This is where, in our yoga, the very practical merges with the deeply spiritual.

Nowhere in the practice of yoga does this meeting of the practical and the spiritual become more real than in the practice of Ahimsa, the practice of non-violence. Through non-violence this meeting of the practical and the spiritual becomes very real both in our practice on our mats and when we take our yoga out into our world. And in the India of old they say Ahimsa Paramo Dharma.[23] Which essentially means *'non-violence is the highest dharma'.* Now dharma is used in several contexts: often in yoga, and as we saw in the previous chapter, it is used in the sense of duty as in Arjuna's duty as a warrior.[24] And it is used in the sense of teaching, as the Buddhists use it to refer to the teachings of the Buddha.

There is however a deeper meaning to dharma: that which supports. In this sense non-violence becomes the way of connecting with that which supports everything. To use the Taoist terminology the practice of Ahimsa is the practice of the path of least resistance: the practice of connecting with the Tao, with life force, with Prana, or whatever label we care to use. *And to return to our discussion on yoga and codes of ethics, from this perspective the natural order of things is the ethical order of things.* Nature works in perfect balance and flow, and rightness or right action, originates from this balance and flow. Acting in accordance with the natural order of things is ethical action. This is action originating from the wisdom gained from rubbing up against this deeper reality. This acting cannot be codified, it is birthed from experiential wisdom and necessitates navigating real tensions as we engage in life from moment to moment.

So we embrace mystery and we loosen that tight little grip we hold on reality. We let go of the boxes we put things in. Because when we put things in boxes they have this tendency to conform to the box. This is another way of saying that words - the labels we use - grip us in their illusion of power. They exert a pull on us as we create reality from moment to moment. However words cannot bring the unseen to the seen: at most words can help us make sense of the unseen. And making sense of something is not the same as experiencing something. The experience is one thing and the making sense of it is another thing. One becomes two and the captivating game of the One playing with itself begins.

This is a warning we find time and again in the texts from the East and nowhere more succinctly than the opening line of the Tao Te Ching: *'Tao called Tao is not Tao.'*[25] So another way of looking at our yoga as our practice deepens is that we practice no story today. To move beyond story is to move into mystery, and it is to move towards yoga. *This is just another way of saying that we are much more mysterious than we can possibly think we are.* The mystery, the yoga, is beyond mind. And the challenge of moving beyond mind is as simple as it is radical; as confrontational as it is comforting; and as beautiful as it is terrifying.

The Play of Life

As above, so below. In the Hatha Yoga tradition, and other traditions from the ancient East, no distinction is made between outside and inside. This is similar to the Western Hermetic tradition which has as one of its basic principles: as above, so below. Which means firstly that the defining characteristics of above are those of below. Secondly, and going further, this means that in reality as the world we find our selves in there is no line demarking above and below, no line demarking outside and inside. As the yogis of old put it: we are all One. Or as the scientist of the modern world put it: all arises from, and returns to, a mysterious field of energy. As is, reality is one, and is all engaged in the endless play of life in balance and flow.

However in a very practical sense we are obliged to use demarcation lines to structure, communicate, and act in the world we find our selves in. In this sense these lines serve us as we manifest on the stage of life in the here and now. This manifestation flows from a sense of purpose that stems from connection with that space inside that is the space outside. From this perspective manifestation from lines is the burden that comes with that connection that is the blessing of yoga. So whilst we use our lines, we do this with the glint of spirit in our eyes, and we acknowledge that a line is just a line.

The most ubiquitous line that we draw in the proverbial sand is one of inside and outside: the line that originates from the belief of separation as me and not-me. This line, when it hardens and solidifies forms a kink, then a twist, then a knot. This knot then distorts and, as it grows, blocks the balance and flow of life in doing its thing. In this way the belief in separation becomes in the world of connection a destructive belief and one that leads to all sorts of problems. In particular this belief manifests as the disembodiment we experience within our selves and that we see in the world around us. This disembodiment is a direct consequence of a hardening of this line of separation. To soften this line, to ground our selves in the perspective that a line is just a line, is to restore balance and flow. So let's turn our attention to two qualities that, when it comes to our own experience, pay absolutely no attention to our line of inside and out. These are two qualities whose essence is unchanged whether we look inside or outside and ones we can relate to our simple anatomy of belly, head and heart. Let's turn our attention to work and play, and at how our yoga practice on our mats builds these qualities.

Work and play. Our practice on our mats is a practice of work and play. It is practice for the work and play we engage in when we take our yoga off our mats and into our worlds, where we engage with and within the One playing with it self. *On our mats we work and we play to disentangle from our habitual ways of engagement to come into the here and now.* These habitual ways of engagement are characterised by an inability to pay attention or maintain focus to the here and now. They are characterised by a dashing from one thing to the next driven by our likes and dislikes, when we are driven by a belief that this thing, that thing, and always the next thing, is going to take us to the place of our heart's fulfilment.

Our practice on our mats is work. Our practice is a desire in our hearts to effect change, translated to intent in our heads, and manifested as action of belly on our mats. It requires building the discipline to roll out our mats for practice. This is a dedication to our practice that we build over time through intention manifested in this action repeated. It also requires growing our ability to focus staying with and within our practice and whatever our practice brings: a focus on being in, and accepting, the here and now. And for the vast majority of us building discipline and growing our ability to focus feels like work.

Our practice on our mats is also play. However, rather than the common manifestation of play as competition this is pure play. It is play for the sake of play. This play is open-ended, where we engage without attachment to outcome. It is play where we are totally captivated by what we are engaged in. In this play we are totally focused, time stands still, and we are one with the play in the here and now. And this play brings us - in and of itself - to a place of pure enjoyment. Our hearts open and we access that place of unbridled happiness inside. The illustration below illustrates balance and flow of work and play across our belly, head and heart.

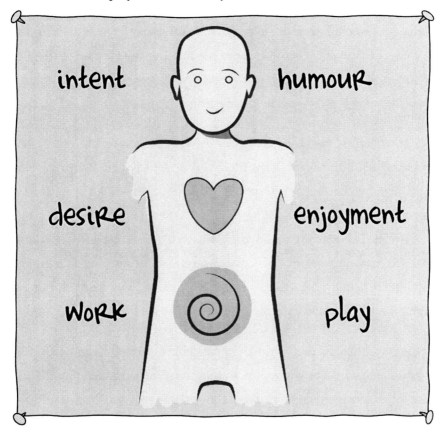

The power of play in our practice is that play picks us up and takes us places - places in the here and now. Places we did not envisage being taken to when we rolled out our mats. At times play picks us up and takes us softly and at times we get caught up in a whirlwind. So one perspective for our practice on our mats is that of a never-ending dance of work and play. A dance where ultimately play trumps work every time, although it may not always seem that way. The never-ending dance of work and play is a perspective that we take off our mats into our worlds.

The metaphor of our practice as play goes a lot deeper than belly, head and heart. Firstly because when we take our yoga off our mats we are invited to entertain the idea that the metaphor of playing games on the stage of life is much more apt than one of walking paths, or in many cases 'working' paths. And secondly because as our practice deepens the persona we put on as we take to this stage becomes more porous. This porosity allows the light of our spirit to shine through in all we do. So in this sense the metaphor of work and play is an invitation to get spiritual.

Get spiritual! Some *thinkers* of the West - in particular in the reductionist and materialist traditions - have tried, and ultimately failed, to destroy our connection with spirit. Because the line we have drawn in the sand is not just one that separates each of us from each other, it is one that separates us from spirit. The world of separation then says: across this line you will not cross. At least not here and not now - wait until you are dead. It is time for us to get spiritual again. Get spiritual in whatever way works for us and from a perspective of connection.

Getting spiritual in the world of connection is very different to getting spiritual in a world of separation. Getting spiritual in the world of balance and flow is a very different proposition to getting spiritual in a world where all plays out to plan. In the old world, plan at the world level plays out in the idea of destiny at an individual level. And we get stuck with questions about our destiny. *In the mysterious world of balance and flow there is no destiny to ask a question about.* In other words, in the world of separation destiny is a manifestation of the getting there red herring - a mechanism to keep us in our box. When we practice yoga in a way that is both radical and simple we acknowledge the power and primacy of mystery.

One key point about mystery is that mystery is a very different thing to mystique. One of the things that traditions do - both in yoga and more broadly - is they replace mystery with mystique. Mystique is slippery and essentially functions, or acts, as a smokescreen, between the One and us. The traditions then jump in and offer - when we follow their teachings, their Dharma - to remove that smokescreen. This is the same smokescreen that they just erected or the illusion that they have put before us. Traditions often dangle carrots as moving targets just beyond our reach.

Mystery, on the other hand, is something we can all engage with directly. Mystery is something we can embrace with our whole being. Ultimately, and right towards the end of the Bhagavad Gita, Krishna invites Arjuna to *'give up all Dharma and come to me.'* To drop all teachings, drop all stories. Krishna invites Arjuna to step into the mysterious place from which wisdom flows, purposeful action arises, and heart opens. Krishna invites Arjuna to then act from this place: action that is a purposeful directional thrust that flows from the morality found in the natural order of things. Krishna's invitation to Arjuna, to all of us, is one of acting from this mystery: or more accurately put, to act from the wisdom gained through touching this mystery.

When we move beyond the smokescreens of tradition we discover that yoga is both very radical and very simple. We focus on growing our awareness, we focus on asking questions of - and exploring purpose in - the mystery, we allow our selves to surrender to what is. And through this we grow our experiential wisdom and we realise self-responsibility. We grow the alignment of our actions with the nature of the mystery of self. So yoga when practiced in a way that is both radical and simple is a political - or rather a politically disruptive - act.

Our yoga wakes us up in a way that is intensely political. It wakes us up not in the old sense of the party politics of left or right, liberal or conservative, but in a new sense that is exquisitely personal. Yoga practice brings all kinds of stuff into the light - our physical and emotional addictions, our deepest fears and desires, and the thoughts and energetic patterns that have a hold on us. Yoga works its subtle magic, and brings us to the only two questions that really matter. The two questions at the centre of a new grassroots politics of wholeness: *'who am I?'* and *'how am I going to spend my time here?'*

This is the questioning - the waking up - that beats the heart of what our big shift is all about. It is the questioning at the heart of the agency challenge our world faces. And as we get radical, as we get down to the roots of these questions, we work things out for our selves. Or in other words we cannot reclaim our agency, our birthright with an externally imposed idea of destiny or set of rules. This is an immediate and real consequence of our focus on experience-based wisdom. We resist buying into dogma, we question and we explore. We explore our experience, we explore our beliefs, and we explore the relationship between the two.

And when it comes to this book, or any book, all of this comes down to: read the book and absorb with your whole being the information that speaks to you. Then let it go. Do your practice and let your whole life be your practice. Know that structure is just structure, that frameworks are just frameworks. And know that you can let go of structure at any time. This is to say that embracing freedom - and getting spiritual - in the connected world comes at a price. And that price is an ever loosening from the grip of inherited mind maps and an ever growing assuming of our own agency in mystery. Embracing the mystery beyond mind is yoga made real in action.

Inner Prop: Embrace Mystery

The Prop: Growing our ability to embrace mystery starts with letting go of knowing mind. When we let go of knowing mind we embrace the unknown and we start to explore. Because it is exploration, and emphatically not knowing, that is the flip side of ignorance. And to explore we engage in play, a very specific sort of play. A play that is both purposeful and purposeless. A play that is a compliment to and ultimately trumps our work of focus.

The mystery is in the ordinary - this is one very important message given to us by the Taoist worldview, the worldview of the One playing in an endless dance of life. Mystery is right under our noses in our own experience. It is in our experience of what is going on inside, in our immediate environment, in our experience of time and space. *And the really juicy thing about mystery is we can get real up close and intimate with mystery, here and now.* There is no holy grail hidden behind a veil that only a select few are allowed to peer behind.

Play in an interconnected and mysterious world - one whose basic qualities are balance and flow - is a very different invitation to play on the stage of isolated objects doing their thing in space and time. The purpose of this play is to engage with and from this deeper reality; the purposelessness of this play is that we engage for the sake of engagement. The seemingly oxymoronic consequence of this purposeless engagement is that it - in and of itself - brings us to a place of a deeper sense of purpose. And, as we will discover, we get fulfilment and pure joy thrown in for good measure.

The Prop of Mystery on our Mats: Our mat-based yoga practice is one of embracing the unknown rather than clinging to the known. This is the invitation presented to us early on in our yoga practice when we - irrespective of our initial motivations for practice - start to see things about ourselves and about yoga that we did not envisage when we started out. We experience that, in taking up the practice of yoga, we have stepped into something much bigger and much more mysterious than we thought we had when we started out.

The invitation to embrace the unknown plays out on our mats from many perspectives. It plays out from the perspective of our physical bodies in the exploration of embodying each posture as we practice - embodiment in the here and now. This embodiment is not the embodiment of yesterday, not the embodiment of tomorrow, and nor is it the embodiment of our fellow yoga practitioners. Our embracing of the unknown plays out in our exploration - and in the endless figuring out - of this embodiment. It is endless simply because we can never embody the same posture twice.

It plays out from the perspective of our belly, head and hearts, as we practice on our mats to connect and explore balance in our observing, feeling and doing. It plays out in the ever deepening merging with the balance and flow of being that is the mystery called spirit. *Through the practice of yoga on our mats we open to realise that we are much more mysterious than we can possibly think we are.* This is moving beyond knowing mind made real.

And it plays out from the perspective of dissolving into the mystery of breath: into the breath that is life force moving in and out of us, that moves us beyond the limited world of our senses, and that links us to the web of life and the realm of spirit. It plays out from the perspective of both the breath that we take and the breath that takes us. Because without the breath we take we are no one, and as we dissolve into the breath that takes us we are no one. This is a perspective that softens and fades our hardened worldview of space and time.

In these ways and more our practice of yoga on our mats grows our sense of ease with not knowing. And it is this sense of ease with not knowing, more than the not knowing in itself, that is worth more than its weight in gold. It is this sense of ease that opens our minds, helps us keep an open mind, and opens our hearts to courage and compassion.

The Prop of Mystery in our Worlds: **When we play with the prop of mystery in our worlds we acknowledge the uniqueness of this present moment.** When we really acknowledge, with our whole beings, then from that real acknowledgment starts our engagement in the play of life - or in other words, we step into the unknown to explore. This present moment becomes the simplest, purest, and most powerful of unknowns.

This exploration - this play - like on our mats is both purposeful and purposeless. The purpose of our play in the world is right action, action for the good of all. And the purposelessness of our play is authentic growth and development. This purpose manifests as persona acting with intention filled with the light of spirit as love. This purposelessness recognises the unknowable complexity of the world we step into and explore to navigate right action. This purposelessness acknowledges that the world does not have to play out to plan, that rules are just rules and codes are just codes. Purpose and purposelessness merge as our growth coming from our ability to manifest right action from the tensions inherent in this complexity. Or put another way: we do act with a plan, and we act with the acceptance that our plan can change at any moment.

The feedback we receive from this play in complexity is the beginning and not the end of mystery. It is the beginning of our exploration. This is the delight and the burden that is Karma: because Karma in essence is the One learning from itself. And Karma in essence is our learning to rub up and merge with the One. It is growing our ability to live in harmony with that which supports everything.

7. The Warrior and the Healer

The old world is crumbling and a new one is being born. As warriors and healers we manifest as creativity to make the shift from separation to connection real. We do this from our individuality to the larger whole, each in our own way. To support us in this is yoga's gift now.

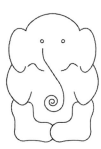

The Call to Arms is the Call to Heal

Our war, our healing. The Bhagavad Gita uses war as the vehicle for its message and Arjuna the warrior as its hero. Arjuna engages in war both inside and out: he engages in war within himself and with his family. Arjuna steps into the unknown with purpose both inside and out to realise the message of the Bhagavad Gita. *And that message, the purpose of his stepping into the unknown, is healing.* This healing very literally involves bringing back together what has been separated into parts. It is a healing that begins on the inside by the realisation of Krishna's message. And it is a healing, in Arjuna's case of the kingdom of Bharat, which he takes to the outside through the action of picking up his arms, his bow and arrows, and taking to the battlefield.

The message of the Bhagavad Gita is as relevant today as it was in Arjuna's time. Make no mistake about it there is a war going on. The old world of separation is no longer serving the whole. This is war that starts as a shift in consciousness and that manifests as, to use that term again, a Great Turning.[26] This is war as manifestation of balance and flow. This is a war between the warrior vanguard of the new world of connection and the temple priests and foot soldiers of the old world of separation. It is a war outside that mirrors, and is mirrored by, our struggle inside. And the warrior vanguard of the world of connection are non-violent, peace-loving, love-loving. They are focused on healing self, community and world.

Our war of worldviews is a war that plays out at many levels. In particular it plays out through patterns of belief, of value, and of system. These three things are of course in the worldview of connection one thing: when we try to draw a line between belief and value, or between value and system, we run up against a wall of impossibility. This is the same wall that we run up against when we practice the yoga of the Yoga Sutras and we try to draw a line between thought and emotion, and emotion and our physical bodies. Patterns of belief bubble up into value patterns that in turn bubble up into system patterns. These are three elements of, or perspectives on, one whole. We are going to look at our war from these three perspectives, and just like our yoga on our mat we'll start with the most visible part of the whole. We'll start with our thicker pieces of rope, our patterns of system, move on to values, then we'll come to the thin strings of belief.

The basic model in the worldview of separation is one of a reality playing out to plan. And playing out to plan brings systems based on command and control. These systems favour hierarchy, they concentrate power, and they strengthen identification with persona. These systems drive the efficiency machine and serve the few rather than the many. They serve the self and not the One. These systems are important because systems, and the context around those systems, play an essential role in shaping our behaviours: in structuring the relationships between individuals and between groups.

When we look at the systems of the world of separation, the systems of the world of mainstream, from the perspective of the new world of connection, what is striking is how often things have been turned the wrong way around. Somewhere along the way we've lost sight of purpose. Purpose has got buried and lost below the burden of system machinery - we just take a look at large swathes of our work in any sector of society and make our own mind up. So what we are seeing in the systems of mainstream is above all a crisis of purpose. The efficiency machine conditions us to focus on asking too often how to do things right, rather than asking what do we want to do. *And, when we ask how to do something right when we are not sure we are doing the right thing, then there is always a hidden assumption.* There is something unseen that constrains us. Asking what we want to do throws the whole thing right open. It necessitates much more creativity than asking how to do things right. However before we get to creativity, we have values and beliefs to look at.

In our separated world we are deeply embedded in systems that we widely acknowledge to be stretched to bursting point. These are systems that from the perspective of the connected world are not fit for purpose. This brings us to patterns of value. *Because in the unseen, in the hidden assumptions and the dislocation with purpose, lie patterns of value.* And our war is also a war of values. The world of separation values amassing stuff, it values material wealth and the consumption of endless bits and pieces. In contrast the world of connection values well-being, it values contentment in wholeness. The world of separation values extraction, the value that breeds the *'what can I get'* mindset. The world of connection values creation, it births the *'what can I contribute'* mindset. The world of separation values individual power, whereas the world of connection values community and love.

Again there is nothing right or wrong here, nothing wrong with either pattern of value. Our war is not a blame game. There was a time when the values of separation served us, otherwise we would not have adopted and acted on them. The systems we built from these values worked for the whole for a while. But what works, and however well it works, also contains the seed of its own decay. This is yin and yang in action in balance and flow. That time of decay is now: these values are not working for us now, they are no longer useful now that the game is changing. And value systems follow from belief systems: at its most fundamental level our war is a war of beliefs.

A new holy trinity? **What we believe in are our gods. Our beliefs play into our values and systems.** Our beliefs drive our behaviour and in a very real sense they rule our world. Casting our mind back to Chapter Two, the message of science and yoga is both clear and radically simple: a god we have worshipped down the ages, the god of separation, is dead. This god of separation comes - as we have seen - with the two sidekicks of inadequacy and disempowerment. The second message we are getting from both West and East is that there is a mysterious energy field or life force that is the source of everything. And that everything includes each and every one of us. We, as conscious human individuals working and playing in this material work, emerge and return to this field. As energy charges or energy bodies we never left it: we have always been, and always will be, an intimate part of the whole. At this level we are in contact with everything that ever has been and ever will be. At this level we are perfect. We are all. *Again the message of science and of yoga is radically simple: it is also time to bury the sidekicks of inadequacy and disempowerment.*

There are three ways we can respond to this message. Firstly, we can reject it. We can respond along the lines of: this is just philosophical abstraction and at most it is a level of truth that does not have any significance for me and my life. Secondly, we can accept it without questioning. This response risks reducing the message to a new-age catchphrase: the message becomes something static or dead and that has little chance of bubbling up to infuse our being and doing. The third response is we can explore it: *we can rise to the individual challenge to actualise this message in our way, and to a degree that works for us wherever we are, in our own being and doing. We can rise to the call to arms that is the call to healing.*

When we need a new Holy Trinity it is this: connection comes with abundance and empowerment. To explore connection we trust - we have faith - in abundance and we embrace empowerment. We face up to our deeply engrained patterns of fear and laziness. We play our part in making the consciousness shift real through self-realisation. We practice the yoga of going inside, of exploring our inner world, and of going out, of manifesting it in the world. And when we work inside and out to explore connection, abundance and empowerment, we activate a virtuous circle. This is the virtuous circle that moves us towards a deeper sense of purpose and realisation of that purpose. This is the yoga of personal evolution, of change, of simple yet radical change. And the yoga of change necessitates creativity, the fruits of which can manifest in all walks of life.

Become creativity. We tend to box creativity in. We live in a culture that positions creativity as something exclusive to a lucky few: a gift blessed upon artists, writers, those in the performing arts. In this way creativity becomes something they have and we do not. To reposition our perspective on creativity we take a radically simple approach, and we go back to the roots. To create is simply to cause something to exist: anything and not just a work of art, a novel or a performance of dance. *In a very real way yoga as self-actualisation is original and intimate personal creativity.* The practice of yoga is practice in the art of living. It is the art of participating fully in life as creation, creation that starts on the inside and ripples out. And the practice of yoga as the art of living gifts us the ultimate freedom. This is a very different type of freedom to the often-used sense of freedom from something. *Yoga gifts us the freedom to become.*

Yoga does this by bringing the unseen into the seen. In doing so we come to a point where we have the opportunity to cast off the chains that bind us. At the most fundamental level we have an opportunity to dream, to re-imagine, to change the beliefs that drive us. To take this opportunity is to take a step into the unknown, a step that necessitates taking a purposeful risk. It is to take a step into the new, into creation. As warriors we expose our selves to loss; as healers our purpose is growing wholeness. As warriors and healers we take our step and we ride the speed bumps along the way.

We are designed for creativity and the only crux is that each of us has to take this step for our selves - we all take this step on our own. By taking this step we shift from living through suppression and control, and we start to embrace and evolve. We jump into the flow, and we create ripples and we create waves. We grow our engagement with the fullness of life. This is our yoga rising. And once our yoga starts rising we will not want to fall back. We won't want to put the genie back in the bottle.

Leaderless Evolution

Resilience, resilience, resilience! Resilience is our ability to return to balance after being knocked off-kilter, and resilience is our ability to remain in a state of balance as flow whilst the world goes about doing its thing all around us. Resilience is popular right now: it is a buzzword in organisational strategy, in what is euphemistically called human resource management, and in the self-help movement. This is as good a sign as any that our big shift is starting to manifest in many, and sometimes unexpected, places. Resilience is founded on strength and flexibility, and on our ability to find balance and flow in and between strength and flexibility.

Yoga is an original and exquisitely powerful system for building resilience. Yoga is powerful in this respect because the practices of yoga build resilience at all levels. In our Asana practice we are continually faced with coming to a sense of ease in situations that are challenging to say the least. *When we embrace this challenge our yoga builds resilience at the physical level, it builds resilience at the level of our belly, head and heart, and it builds spiritual resilience.* The resilience we get from the practice of yoga is one of yoga's most powerful hooks: one of the reasons yoga works for so many and brings us back to practice.

The very direct way the practice of yoga builds resilience is at the level of our physical body. We build more physical strength and we gain physical flexibility. We become able to hold postures that we find tiring or challenging for longer and with more ease. We find our selves able to embody postures that previously we could not figure. This, for many practitioners of yoga, is the immediate observable effect of Asana practice. We build healthy bodies; we build a strong and flexible physical home.

Yoga also builds resilience at the level of our basic anatomical framework of belly, head and heart. It builds resilience in our centres of doing, observing and feeling within our physical home. In our belly we develop strength and softness of will to action. We cultivate the wisdom and discernment of our belly: we reconnect with, and can better listen to, our gut feelings. In our head we develop wisdom and humour in observation, and we cultivate strength and flexibility in our imagination, in our dreaming. And we grow truth, compassion and passion of heart. The practice of yoga builds all these things and more, and it builds them in its own sweet way.

Yoga builds resilience of spirit through strength and flexibility in our directional thrust of purpose, through growing our ability to both influence the flow and go with it. Ultimately our yoga grows our acceptance of, and surrender to, what is. We grow our sense of ease with whatever is happening, inside and out; we grow our ability to return to our grounding in breath, to deepen our sense of wholeness right now. We start to acknowledge and realise the perfection that is. We grow our ability to embrace each and every moment. *This spiritual resilience is full-power resilience.*

Growing resilience on our mats grows our resilience in our worlds. We grow strength and flexibility - of body and mind, of doing and being. As we grow our resilience, we take courage in action, and we let go of fear and laziness: in a very tangible and powerful way we free our selves from those endemic patterns of fear and laziness in our worlds. And we open our hearts to deep engagement, to our engagement with authentic experience.

From resilience engagement. Resilience is the foundation for full engagement: it provides the strength and flexibility in balance and flow that is the foundation for personal evolution. When we engage from a position of weak resilience we are going to get knocked down. This is often what lies behind yoga injury on our mats - we succumb to the pattern of engagement as striving and we push our selves. We very literally run away with our ego and that gets us into trouble. Engagement from weak resilience is engagement from a position of misalignment. When our desire in our hearts or our intention in our heads are out of whack with the strength and flexibility of our bodies. We take a step too far, a step that is not purposeful, a risk that is not appropriate.

When we engage from a position of relatively strong resilience we are going to get knocked down less often and when we get knocked down we are going to get back up more easily. And what we take from those knockdowns will be different. On our mats we may still incur physical injury but our perspective on injury changes. We shift from injury as hell, to injury as every cloud has a silver lining, and then to the cloud is the silver lining. On and off our mats we get up wiser and richer. We get wiser and richer from loss as we shed illusion.

When we practice yoga on our mats we use method to build resilience and we engage *with* yoga through method. There are many methods for engaging with yoga: as we saw earlier the Yoga Sutras provide at least three methods. Up front in the first chapter method is broken down into two parts: practice and surrender, or do your work and do it with love.[27] Next, at the start of the second chapter, comes Kriya Yoga where method is broken down into three parts. This is the method we explored in Chapter Three through the lens of our philosophers anatomy of belly, head and heart.[28] And later comes Ashtanga Yoga, where method is broken down into eight parts – the method that is known as the eight limbs of yoga. Whichever method or mix of methods we follow, the explicit purpose of method is to support us engaging with yoga, to move us into the state of yoga.

When we engage in life *from* yoga we engage from that state where we are in, and act from, Oneness. When we move to engaging in life from yoga as Oneness method or technique is of no help. We let go of method and manifest as we are: rather than, for example, doing our work and doing it with love we become love manifesting through action. This is shown in the illustration below.

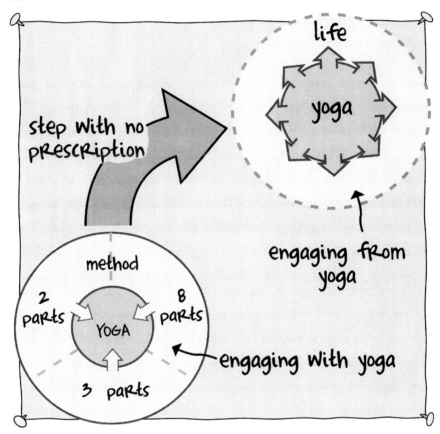

There is no prescription for moving from engaging with yoga through method to engaging in life from yoga. This alone is a very good reason not to get attached to method, not to identify with technique. *Engagement in yoga as life has only one rule: our full participation is required.* Technique and method can get us so far but ultimately we take this step - a step into yoga as creation - on our own, both on our mats and in our worlds.

The shedding of illusion of the refuge of method is the burden of yoga. The richness we realise through shedding this illusion is the blessing of yoga.

These are a burden and a blessing that are both exquisitely intangible and very concrete, both spiritual and practical. These are the burdens and blessings that flow from yoga as a warrior art and yoga as a healing art. Because both the warrior and the healer are at home whether we take the perspective of the world of spirit or the perspective of the world of things. Because the world of spirit is, in connection, the world of things. So when it comes to yoga, radical and simple yoga, the art of the warrior is the art of the healer.

When we engage in our worlds from a position of resilience we each engage in our own way. Just like our yoga as Oneness on our mats, when it comes to manifesting yoga in our worlds we cannot standardise anything of depth. And simply because of the endless diversity of our worlds - and the endless requirements and manifestations of our shift - it means there is space for everyone. There is a role for us each to play. *A role we create through action when we step into leaderless evolution.*[29] When we decide how we are going to spend our time here. When we step into freedom. And as we do so we uncover one of the best kept secrets of all time: *that the security we all yearn for, the sense of peace and of joy, the sense of strength and of purpose, is in the freedom to become.*

When we take either the perspective of the world of spirit or the world of things then engaging from resilience means having strength and flexibility of mind, an open heart, and fire in our belly. Very practically engaging from resilience means leveraging our passions to explore purpose. It means embracing the never-ending learning that comes with deploying our talents. It means stepping beyond pattern and adapting as we learn. And it means acknowledging our individual responsibility and the power of community.

Build community. Arjuna had an army! This is one oft-overlooked element of the Bhagavad Gita: we focus on the hero and we forget that

Arjuna could not do it alone. As we have seen our practices of yoga de-wire us and they rewire us as individuals: when we loosen our selves from our no-longer-useful reactive patterns we very literally rewire our brains. We weaken certain neural nets and create and strengthen new ones. *Our big shift is bringing a de-wiring and rewiring of how we behave together as communities - in our beliefs, our values and our systems.* This is happening at all levels and is a shift in community that is manifesting from collective will built on individual will. When our individual agency bubbles up into collective agency we create the opportunity for larger change.

The thing about leaderless evolution is that to have a crystallised version of what the world of connection will look like at the wider levels of community is at the very least an oxymoron. This uncertainty feeds either our empowerment or our fears. When fear wins out we'll fall back to the old and turn again to systems of suppression and control. And those who tend towards suppression and control have an almost always present tendency to impose this on others. This is not a blame thing - it is just part of the package. Not only do they fear going off the rails themselves, they also fear the embracers of the unknown going off the rails. As our individual work on our mats and in our worlds ripples out we assuage our collective fear. We can come to embody that all we are afraid of has no basis in truth.

The bottom line is we don't know how our big shift is going to develop, how a better world will manifest. Simply put, we don't know whether our big shift will be evolutionary or revolutionary. *Whichever it is, as yogis we bring our non-violence to the table, and we focus on what we do know.* We know that what we do and how we do it matters - this is the experiential wisdom we get from yoga practice. We know that yoga gives us a perspective to take, a lens through which we participate in life: the ever-deepening sense of connection.

We know that the practices of yoga can facilitate our exploration of that something that the metaphors of both ancient East and modern West are rubbing up against: that something from which both our collective interconnectedness and our individual agency are born. We know that our yoga brings the opportunity for transformation, both individually and collectively. This is a transformation that is beyond metaphor and that is grounded directly in the experience of life. And we know we have the courage to resist buying into the values and systems of the age of separation - resist buying into self-centred striving, hierarchy and big leaders.

When it comes to the unknown, to our collective uncertainty in the face of the unknown, our yoga provides the basis for empowerment to win out over fear. Yoga provides the tools - and process - to build sustainable and fulfilling relationships with our selves, those around us, and with the world at large. We know our yoga is getting juicy - that it is beginning to work - when we grow our freedom to be who we really are. And with this freedom comes the space to see others for whom they really are. The space comes to grow authentic relationships with those around us. Or in other words de-wiring community means dissolving the barriers of separation, the separation that starts at home. Reconnection - rewiring - that starts inside, and spreads like ripples on a pond.

This is a grassroots shift and when we look around we see the green shoots of yoga rising everywhere. We see yoga warriors in all walks of life standing up, falling down, and getting up again: yoga warriors playing their part. We see yoga warriors working and playing to shift away from the tradition of hierarchy to reinvent our social and cultural dynamics. For each of us in the yoga community there is no better place to start than at home. Yoga in the West grew big - that is, got the breadth it has today - using the props of the old story: commoditisation, hierarchy, technique and brand. To move collectively towards depth we need to develop a new set of collective props.

Mainstream is crumbling simply because more and more of us are acknowledging that it no longer works. We are recognising that for the most part the institutions and individuals to which we have delegated agency are no longer fit for purpose: they are no longer acting in the interests of our communities or our planet. We are realising that in order to create a better world we have to change something fundamental. We are realising that we have to let go of our belief in separation - of you and me, of us and them, and of humankind and nature. And we are realising that it is time to start acting in the good of the One instead of this one, in the interest of the whole rather than a part. Now is the time to explore that truth yoga has always proclaimed, and that parts of modern science are acknowledging - we are all connected, the ripples and the pond are one.

The house of cards of mainstream is shaking - the old world is dying and a new one is being born. The puppet masters can no longer hide in the shadows. *We are waking up and claiming the space not just to dream but to become. We are cutting the strings, and reclaiming our agency.* We are rising to our unfilled potential. And for those who catch and play on the wave it is one hell of a ride. A ride, or engagement with life, with reality as it unfolds, that deepens as we activate the virtuous circle of the attitude props of yoga. Engagement with life fully now is yoga made real in action.

Inner Prop: Become Creativity

We are born to wake up. We are born to think and to feel in freedom, and from authenticity. We are born to surrender into spontaneity, born to exercise agency through action. And when it comes to creativity for the good of all there are no rules - no fixed codes and no paths for us to walk along. There are no rules as to how and to in what form. When there is a rule it is this: the time is now. Because exercising agency in the now is creativity in action.

Creativity flows effortlessly when we grow the six previous skills, when they merge in subtle ways to become one. To return to the warning given at the end of Chapter One: the one that is aware is not our true self. This misconception is the ultimate commoditisation of the message of yoga. This is separation dressed in the garbs of spiritual materialism. Through yoga we experience that body and soul are one; that what connects us is part of us.

So we let go of a fixed idea or goal of our true self and be true to our self. *When we create from moment to moment using the full awareness available to us then we are being true to our self.* To create in the world of connection is to manifest our humaneness. It is to deviate from the trajectory laid out in the worldview that believes that reality plays out according to plan. *To create in the world of connection is to rise to the potential of our birthright.*

Notes

1. This term 'fruits of our actions' is used repeatedly in the Bhagavad Gita where Krishna instructs Arjuna in yoga.

2. Material excerpted from the book *Tao Te Ching* © 1993 Stephen Addiss & Stanley Lombardo, Hackett Publishing Company Inc.

3. The sentiment expressed by Aristotle has been echoed by modern Western minds as diverse as Benjamin Franklin, George Gurdjieff and Aldous Huxley.

4. See for example the article Hearing The Call by Joanna Macy, *Resurgence & Ecologist*, Issue 277, March/April 2013.

5. The Mahabharata is one of the two epic ancient Indian tales - the other being the Ramayana.

6. When we define yoga as in essence an inner practice then we have to regard studies based on observations of subjects from the outside with a healthy dose of scepticism.

7. From Mahatma Gandhi's speech at Kingsley Hall, London, October 1931.

8. The Hard Problem is essentially one of why we have subjective conscious experience and has been recognized as such for a long time.

9. A Dantian - often spelt Tan Tien - is an energy centre, and Dantian in the singular usually refers to the lower centre that is considered the foundation.

10. Plato proposed his three-part idea of the human soul in *The Republic*.

11. Samadhi is the eighth and final limb in the Ashtanga yoga system presented in the Yoga Sutras. The state of Samadhi is characterised by a still – or undisturbed – mind; a deep meditative state where the mind is concentrated and at one with the object of meditation.

12. Material excerpted from the book *Tao Te Ching* © 1993 Stephen Addiss & Stanley Lombardo, Hackett Publishing Company Inc.

13. This is a broadly used framework for understanding our habitual reactions and behaviours. The terminology trigger, filter & state is taken from *Shine - How to Survive and Thrive at Work* by Chris Barez-Brown, Penguin, 2012.

14. The Yoga Sutras offer at least three methods, or perhaps better put, three perspectives on method. As we move through the text the perspective on method becomes more detailed, offering more structure for the reader. Method is broken down first into two, then three, then finally eight parts.

15. For the translations of both Sutra II-46 and II-47 the material is excerpted from the book *Yoga Sutras of Patanjali* ©2002 Mukunda Stiles, with permission

from Red Wheel/Weiser, LLC Newburyport, MA and San Francisco, CA, www. redwheelweiser.com.

16. I first heard this formulation used by Mark Whitwell in a workshop given in The Netherlands in 2008 and it has stuck with me ever since.

17. This is a reformulation of the first line of the Serenity Prayer by Reinhold Niebuhr, which has been used by Alcoholics Anonymous and other 12-step programmes. The essence of this line has existed in oral form for much longer.

18. This is one of the underlying principles of all forms of yoga practice, both those focusing on the physical and energetic bodies and the yoga of the Bhagavad Gita.

19. The five quotes related to myth are excerpted from the book *A Short History of Myth* © 2005 Karen Armstrong, with permission from Canongate Books Ltd.

20. These three points are distilled from the excellent and broad-ranging book on warriorship *The Craft of the Warrior*, Robert L. Spencer, North Atlantic Books

21. Yoga as skill in action is one of many definitions of yoga given to Arjuna by Krishna in the Bhagavad Gita. Skill in action essentially refers to our ability to intentionally impact the world around us.

22. This definition of risk is taken from *Risk Thinking*, Ralph Coverdale and published by Coverdale, 1977.

23. This often-quoted saying comes from the Mahabharata.

24. For Arjuna, as a warrior trained in the arts of war, the line immediately following the line 'non-violence is the highest dharma' was just as pertinent: 'So too is violence in the service of dharma.'

25. See Note 2. above.

26. See Note 4. above.

27. This is analogous to the teachings of the modern Indian spiritual teacher Neem Karoli Baba: Love All, Serve All.

28. This is analogous to the teachings of another modern Indian spiritual teacher Babaji, or Haidakhan Babaji: Truth, Love, Simplicity.

29. This phrase was inspired by the title of the excellent book *Leaderless Revolution* by Carne Ross.

Acknowledgements

I bow deeply to the practices of yoga which came into my life more than 15 years ago and have been a source of exploration and inspiration ever since. I offer my thanks to all the gifted teachers I have had the opportunity to work and play with over the years, in particular: Gösta Van Dam and Patrick Vermeulen of Svaha Yoga Amsterdam for opening my eyes and spirit to the fullness of yoga; Mark Whitwell whose masterful transmission of the simplicity of the teachings of yoga went straight to my heart; Nicole Aarons for the off-the-wall shamanic wildness in my early years of practice; Simona Hernandez of Yoga Bodhi in Bath for the impeccable technical guidance; Radha and Pierre of Yoga Plus in Crete where I have been a guest for many years; and the Barefoot Doctor for imparting Taoist magic.

I am deeply grateful to all who have played a role in making this book happen: to Josie Sykes, Karen Whitfield and Moira Goulmy for feedback on early drafts; to Eva Thomassen for the beautiful Ganesh illustration used on the cover; to Chris Kerslake for transforming my sketches for the interior illustrations into legible art work; and to Saijdah Saleem for proof reading the final draft. Any remaining errors or unintelligible utterances are of course my responsibility. I also thank the whole team at EkhartYoga for giving me the space to offer videos and blogs through the EkhartYoga site; to Elephant Journal and to Sharda Devika for posting a few of my articles when I was starting to put pen to paper back in 2012 and 2013; and to the hundreds of people I have worked with either individually or in group settings as a coach and trainer.

I pay tribute to my family and friends: to my mother for her loving acceptance of whatever the next unexpected step was that I took through the years; to my father for transmitting a little of his curiosity and the importance of never giving up in the face of our work to see through the smokescreens that cover so much of our modern world; to my sisters Eleanor and Sue simply for being sisters. To Tom Low, Chris Taylor, Bas Ruyssenaars, Ingrid van Gestel, Moira Goulmy, Kate Gould, Anne Walsh, Elmar Fritsch, Cristina Vano, Dirk-Jan de Vink, José de Groot, Josie Sykes, Isabel Watson and Sarah Garrett – for friendships that have stood the test of time, and enriched my life in immeasurable and exquisitely different ways.

To my partner Judi: writing for me was often *'cave work'* - thank you for respecting this and for the warmth each time I emerged. Exploring and riding the balance and flows of our relationship has taught me more about yoga than any book or the formal practices of yoga on my mat. To Honey - our cat - or rather the little being in a cat outfit who hangs out at our place: whilst Honey may not be the best in accepting the closed door of the cave, she has shown endless patience in demonstrating the art of *Wu Wei*.

Lightning Source UK Ltd.
Milton Keynes UK
UKOW04f0026110316

270007UK00004B/217/P